Living with Tinnitus

Laurence McKenna, M. Clin. Psychol., PhD, qualified as a clinical psychologist from the University of Liverpool in 1983. He also trained in cognitive behaviour therapy at the University of Oxford. He has worked as a clinical psychologist at the Royal National Throat Nose & Ear Hospital for the past 27 years. He is head of the team of psychologists working in the Adult Audiological Medicine Department treating patients with tinnitus and other audiovestibular disorders. He is an honorary lecturer at the Ear Institute (UCL) and honorary visiting fellow at the University of Bristol.

Laurence is the author or co-author of many academic papers, chapters and a book on tinnitus and other aspects of psychology and audiological medicine. He is a member of the professional advisory committee of the British Tinnitus Association and was co-director of the European Tinnitus Course for seven years.

David Baguley, BSc, MSc, MBA, PhD, is Director of Audiology at Cambridge University Hospitals, UK. David's clinical and research interests focus on tinnitus, with the aim of understanding this symptom and designing novel and innovative interventions.

His initial studies were at the University of Manchester, in psychology and then clinical audiology. He has a PhD in the subject of tinnitus from the University of Cambridge. He has authored many papers and co-authored several books. In 2006 David received an International Award in Hearing from the American Academy of Audiology and has twice been awarded the Shapiro Prize from the British Tinnitus Association for tinnitus research (2005, 2008).

David is a Fellow at Wolfson College, Cambridge, and is a Visiting Professor at Anglia Ruskin University.

Don McFerran is a consultant ear, nose and throat surgeon in the UK's oldest town, Colchester. Don has worked as an ENT surgeon since 1983 and has had a specific interest in tinnitus since 1987, when he trained under Jonathan Hazell.

Don is the author or co-author of numerous scientific articles, book chapters and a book on tinnitus. He has also been one of the co-directors of the European Tinnitus Course since 2005 and is currently Chair of the Professional Advisers' Committee to the British Tinnitus Association.

Overcoming Common Problems Series

Selected titles

A full list of titles is available from Sheldon Press,
36 Causton Street, London SW1P 4ST and on our website at
www.sheldonpress.co.uk

Asperger Syndrome in Adults
Dr Ruth Searle

The Assertiveness Handbook
Mary Hartley

Assertiveness: Step by step
Dr Windy Dryden and Daniel Constantinou

Backache: What you need to know
Dr David Delvin

Body Language: What you need to know
David Cohen

The Cancer Survivor's Handbook
Dr Terry Priestman

The Chronic Fatigue Healing Diet
Christine Craggs-Hinton

The Chronic Pain Diet Book
Neville Shone

Cider Vinegar
Margaret Hills

The Complete Carer's Guide
Bridget McCall

Confidence Works
Gladeana McMahon

Coping Successfully with Pain
Neville Shone

Coping Successfully with Period Problems
Mary-Claire Mason

Coping Successfully with Prostate Cancer
Dr Tom Smith

Coping Successfully with Psoriasis
Christine Craggs-Hinton

Coping Successfully with Ulcerative Colitis
Peter Cartwright

Coping Successfully with Varicose Veins
Christine Craggs-Hinton

Coping Successfully with Your Hiatus Hernia
Dr Tom Smith

Coping Successfully with Your Irritable Bowel
Rosemary Nicol

Coping When Your Child Has Cerebral Palsy
Jill Eckersley

Coping with Age-related Memory Loss
Dr Tom Smith

Coping with Birth Trauma and Postnatal Depression
Lucy Jolin

Coping with Bowel Cancer
Dr Tom Smith

Coping with Candida
Shirley Trickett

Coping with Chemotherapy
Dr Terry Priestman

Coping with Chronic Fatigue
Trudie Chalder

Coping with Coeliac Disease
Karen Brody

Coping with Compulsive Eating
Dr Ruth Searle

Coping with Diabetes in Childhood and Adolescence
Dr Philippa Kaye

Coping with Diverticulitis
Peter Cartwright

Coping with Eating Disorders and Body Image
Christine Craggs-Hinton

Coping with Epilepsy in Children and Young People
Susan Elliot-Wright

Coping with Family Stress
Dr Peter Cheevers

Coping with Gout
Christine Craggs-Hinton

Coping with Hay Fever
Christine Craggs-Hinton

Coping with Headaches and Migraine
Alison Frith

Coping with Hearing Loss
Christine Craggs-Hinton

Coping with Heartburn and Reflux
Dr Tom Smith

Coping with Kidney Disease
Dr Tom Smith

Coping with Life after Stroke
Dr Mareeni Raymond

Overcoming Common Problems Series

Overcoming Common Problems Series

Overcoming Common Problems

Living with Tinnitus and Hyperacusis

DR LAURENCE McKENNA,
DR DAVID BAGULEY and
DR DON McFERRAN

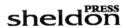
sheldon PRESS

First published in Great Britain in 2010

Sheldon Press
36 Causton Street
London SW1P 4ST
www.sheldonpress.co.uk

British Library Cataloguing-in-Publication Data
A catalogue record for this book is available from the British Library

ISBN 978-1-84709-083-6

1 3 5 7 9 10 8 6 4 2

Typeset by Fakenham Photosetting Ltd, Fakenham, Norfolk
Printed in Great Britain by Ashford Colour Press

Produced on paper from sustainable forests

This book is dedicated to Nancy and Brian McFerran, Anne O'Sullivan, and Sam, Naomi and Luke Baguley

Contents

Foreword

'Is there a cure for tinnitus?'

As the former national chairman of the American Tinnitus Association, and as the organizer of my own city tinnitus support group, this is usually the first question from anybody who suddenly finds themselves with weird and disagreeable sounds in their ears. General practitioners, audiologists, and ears, nose and throat doctors hear this question all the time too. Many of these health-care workers unfortunately answer the question the wrong way. 'No,' they say brusquely, 'there isn't. You will just have to go home and learn to live with it.'

The authors of *Living with Tinnitus and Hyperacusis* answer the question the *right* way. Through long years of professional clinical experience and psychological therapeutic practice, they recognize the anxiety and hopelessness underlying the question. And they offer a remarkable response. Whether or not the sound of tinnitus can be eradicated is still an open issue subject to ongoing research, but what is clear is that you don't have to allow it to affect your quality of life. And by choosing not to let tinnitus, and its related condition hyperacusis, adversely affect you, they will no longer be issues.

How can the authors make such a claim? They first explain the complex auditory and neurological causes for tinnitus, having learned from their research and clinical practices that the more you know about tinnitus, the more empowered you are to neutralize it. They show what to expect during the standard medical treatment protocols. The fact that these tests find *nothing wrong* with the patients in the overwhelming majority of cases should not be a cause for despair, they say – it is instead a cause for relief that no health-threatening condition has to be confronted. Using helpful diagrams and checklists, they reveal the underlying psychological conditions that predispose some people to tinnitus – and how those can be countered. Medications, sleep, the baffling array of other symptoms that sometimes accompany tinnitus, the latest medical research – this book covers the full spectrum of the experience of tinnitus and hyperacusis, and how you can help yourself with clinically proven approaches.

So if you have just acquired tinnitus, and don't know what to do – this book is for you. If you have suffered with this debilitating condition for many years and still find yourself grasping for some relief (the 'eternal quest', as the authors call it) – this book is for you. If somebody you know and care about is going through the torment of this invisible malady – this book is for you. There are almost as many books on tinnitus out there as there are bogus quack remedies – but this is one book that I would not hesitate to highly recommend on a personal basis to my own friends with tinnitus.

Scott C. Mitchell
Former Chairman of the Board of Directors
American Tinnitus Association

Preface

There is no doubt that tinnitus can be a terrible affliction, not only for the affected individual but also for friends and family. The prospects for recovery, however, have never been better, thanks to new scientific understanding and approaches to therapy. There is a tremendous ongoing effort to identify treatments and therapies that will inhibit tinnitus, but many people are left to fend for themselves.

In this book, we seek to lay out the strategies and tactics for dealing with troublesome tinnitus that we have found to be effective, in the hope that they will allow those who are not presently finding accessible and effective tinnitus treatment to improve their situation and quality of life.

Note to the reader

This is not a medical book and is not intended to replace advice from your doctor. Consult your doctor if you believe you have any of the symptoms described and if you think you might need medical help.

Part 1
DEFINING THE PROBLEM

1

Introduction and definitions

Tinnitus is one of the commonest physical symptoms affecting humanity. Despite this fact, it is only in recent years that our understanding of tinnitus has really progressed.

Although most people have heard of tinnitus, this probably explains why very few of us have any real understanding of this common symptom. The confusion extends to both the spelling and pronunciation of tinnitus. In the UK, the word is correctly pronounced as *tin-it-us*, though the American pronunciation *ti-night-us* is also acceptable.

Tinnitus can be defined as the conscious awareness of a sound sensation that is not due to an external sound source. As we shall see later, however, even producing a definition is not straightforward and there are various different definitions and subgroups. Although many people think of tinnitus as ringing in the ears, a huge variety of sounds can be perceived. These range from single tones to complex, even musical, sounds.

One of the truly curious things about tinnitus is that only a small proportion of people who experience the symptom are significantly upset by it. It is therefore important to make a distinction between simple awareness of tinnitus and the distress that this awareness sometimes produces.

For those who do have distressing tinnitus, the experience can be life-altering. Individuals and families may struggle with sleep, concentration and deeply felt irritability and agitation. In some cases, it seems as if a person has undergone a personality change, becoming fearful and isolated. Such changes, however, are not inevitable and, when they do happen, they need not be permanent. There are well-established paths towards recovery. This may not be an easy journey and some may find that their recovery is not complete, but the central proposition of this book is that recovery from distressing tinnitus is possible and the essential building blocks are straightforward – namely information, sound therapy and relaxation therapy. One framework that interweaves these, with other therapeutic elements, is cognitive behavioural therapy (CBT) and it forms the backbone of this book.

'Why,' you may ask, 'is there no cure? Why does there need to be a book such as this rather than a course of medication or, perhaps, laser treatment?' The reasons are both complex and interesting. Tinnitus has a huge variety of causes and impacts, so it is unlikely that there is a single solution for all these variations. Furthermore, the reaction of the individual is strongly influenced by personality, family and work context so the notion of a one size fits all solution is not realistic.

Although people with distressing tinnitus perceive a sound, the condition often behaves more like a pain, especially in terms of the variety of reactions. In some people, the extent of the distress can lead to depression and severe turbulence, including problems at home and at work. In others, however, it is simply a background sensation that is neither problematic nor intrusive and the distress they feel is minimal.

How does someone move from the troubled state into recovery? This is a question that we will return to.

Definitions

There are many definitions of tinnitus in the scientific literature. Some run to several pages and some are written with large amounts of scientific jargon. There are also, however, some relatively simple and user-friendly descriptions.

In 1982, Dennis McFadden considered tinnitus to be 'the conscious expression of a sound that originates in an involuntary manner in the head of its owner, or may appear to him to do so'. This definition has been widely adopted. It is quite helpful and clear, though some people have tinnitus that appears to be localized outside the head or even elsewhere in the body.

Another simple, accessible definition is offered by Canadian researchers Jos Eggermont and Larry Roberts, who said that tinnitus is 'an auditory phantom sensation (ringing of the ears) experienced when no external sound is present'.

American researcher Carol Bauer described tinnitus as, 'an auditory sensation without an external stimulus.'

Different types of tinnitus and hyperacusis

One distinction that used to be made was that between *subjective* and *objective* tinnitus.

In the subjective category, only the individual affected can hear a sound. With objective tinnitus, the sound can also be heard by someone else – usually with the help of a stethoscope or other amplifying device. In such cases, the sound is being generated physically within the body. These commonly include clicking and awareness of the pulse and are now entitled *somatosounds*, as the body physically creates them. This sort of tinnitus is less common – most people who have tinnitus have the subjective kind. The noise they hear is not generated elsewhere in the body, but is the result of some change in the auditory system.

A symptom often associated with tinnitus is *hyperacusis*, which is a hypersensitivity of hearing. This does not mean the ability to hear extraordinarily quiet sounds like Superman! People with hyperacusis have excessively sensitive hearing and find it difficult to tolerate ordinary day-to-day sounds that most people would regard as quiet or unintrusive. They feel irritated by sound or notice that sounds interfere with their ability to concentrate. A few may experience more significant distress, or even pain, in response to exposure to sounds.

Various studies have shown that most people who have hyperacusis also have tinnitus. If we look at these figures the opposite way round, however, we find that most people who have tinnitus do not also have hyperacusis. It is very difficult to get accurate figures about hyperacusis, but even the most pessimistic survey showed that only about 40 per cent of people with tinnitus reported hyperacusis and other studies gave much lower rates. Whatever the real figures, it is clear that hyperacusis is much less common than tinnitus.

In those cases where tinnitus and hyperacusis exist together, the combination can undoubtedly be troublesome. For some, hyperacusis is the more pressing concern, but for others, the tinnitus is the greater problem. Most hyperacusis is irksome rather than life-changing, though for those with severe hyperacusis, everyday activities can become difficult – the sounds of family life, the washing machine or traffic may be intense and troubling, interfering with their ability to live life to the full. Fortunately, similar strategies can be applied to hyperacusis as are used for tinnitus. That is to say, information, sound therapy, relaxation therapy and CBT can be used to good effect for both.

Historical background to medical knowledge and treatments

It may seem that tinnitus is a problem associated with our noisy modern world. In fact, references to tinnitus have certainly been found right back to antiquity. A series of ancient Babylonian medical texts, inscribed on clay tablets, were contained within the library of King Assurbanipal (668–626 BC) in Nineveh. Translation of these scripts revealed 22 references to tinnitus, described variously as the ears 'singing', 'speaking' or 'whispering'. Treatments are described, including whispered incantations, the instillation of various substances into the external ear canal and the application of charms, such as the tooth of a female ibex.

Tinnitus has six mentions in the *Corpus Hippocratum*, a second-century AD compilation of the works of Hippocrates of Kos (460–377 BC). Other authors writing in Greek and Roman times mentioning tinnitus include Celsus (25 BC – AD 50), who described treatments with diet and abstinence from wine, and Pliny the Elder (AD 23–79), who advocated the use of wild cumin and almond oil in cases of tinnitus.

Little progress was made regarding tinnitus until the eighteenth century, when medical scientist Jean-Marie Itard wrote a textbook on ear disease. Itard noted that troublesome tinnitus can lead to poor sleep and to 'an extremely irksome discomfort which leads to a profound sadness in affected individuals'. He considered the use of sound in managing tinnitus, advising people to live by running water or build up the fire in their grate so that it hissed and popped.

The nineteenth century also saw the rise of otology (the diagnosis and treatment of ear disease) as a distinct medical specialty and two early otologists spent a great amount of time considering tinnitus. The first of these, Joseph Toynbee (1815–66), worked at St Mary's Hospital in London, collecting a large number of medical samples for teaching. Toynbee experienced distressing tinnitus himself and, sadly, died during an experiment in which he attempted to determine 'the effect of inhalation of chloroform upon tinnitus'.

The other early otologist of note was Sir William Wilde (1815–76), father of Oscar Wilde, who wrote extensively on ear disease and described ear conditions that were associated with tinnitus. It was not until 1891, however, that the first book on tinnitus alone, by Henry MacNaughton-Jones, was published.

A major series of advances were made in the 1940s and 1950s in the USA by otologist E. P. Fowler. He worked extensively on tinnitus, at first alone and then with his son, E. P. Fowler Jr, also an otologist, establishing the commonsense groundwork for describing and treating the condition. By this time, electronic advances enabled accurate measurements of hearing, as well as ways of estimating the pitch and intensity of tinnitus.

The work of two pioneers should be acknowledged at this point. Dr Jack Vernon, working at the University of Oregon, pioneered the use of sound therapy and masking devices for tinnitus following discussions with an academic colleague who was so bothered by his tinnitus that he could only concentrate when sitting by a flowing fountain.

Dr Ross Coles, working as an audiological physician in Southampton and Nottingham, investigated medical treatments for tinnitus and worked unceasingly to identify effective therapies. He taught generations of medics and scientists about tinnitus (including us!).

Until relatively recently, this is where the story would have ended. Insights and discoveries from neuroscience, psychology and medicine, however, have led to a far deeper understanding of tinnitus. These understandings will be covered in Part 1, while in Part 2 we shall give you detailed and practical information regarding how to get to grips with tinnitus.

2

The causes of tinnitus and hyperacusis

The question, 'What exactly is causing my tinnitus?' is on the lips of everyone who is distressed by their experiences. In this chapter, we attempt to answer it by describing our model of tinnitus and hyperacusis, which is built on many ideas put forward by people working in this field. We draw, in particular, on the work of Richard Hallam, Ronald Hinchcliffe, Pawel Jastreboff and Jonathan Hazell.

Many theories have attempted to explain tinnitus and hyperacusis. Most focus on defects within the ear, especially the inner ear. Such theories, however, do not explain tinnitus and hyperacusis very effectively. If tinnitus were due simply to damage to the inner ear, how could we explain the fact that many people with tinnitus have normal hearing? Conversely, there are many people with hearing loss who do not have any tinnitus whatsoever.

Hyperacusis is even more difficult to explain in terms of inner ear damage. If the ear is damaged and less information is passing to the brain, how can sounds seem too loud? Common sense would suggest that we would be *less* bothered by sound if our ears were not working properly than more so.

Clearly there must be an explanation and this explanation is, in fact, quite straightforward: the ears are only *part* of the auditory system. To understand tinnitus and hyperacusis, we must consider more of the auditory system and incorporate an understanding of the hearing pathways within the brain – the so-called central auditory system.

Ear anatomy

If you were to look at a diagram of the auditory system in a biology textbook or an encyclopaedia, you would most likely see a diagrammatic representation of the ear rather like that shown in Figure 2.1.

The fleshy outer part of the ear is known as the pinna. This connects, via the ear canal, or external auditory meatus, to the eardrum, or tympanic membrane. The pinna, ear canal and eardrum together constitute the *external ear*.

Outer ear   Middle ear   Inner ear

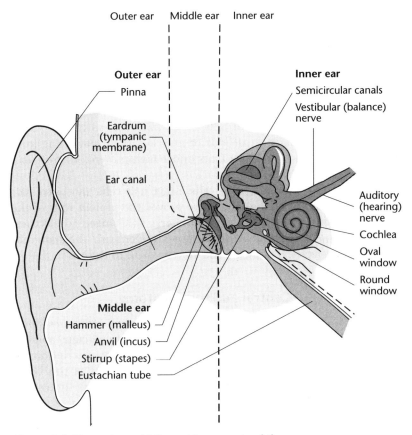

Outer ear
Pinna

Eardrum
(tympanic
membrane)

Ear canal

Inner ear
Semicircular canals
Vestibular (balance)
nerve

Auditory
(hearing)
nerve

Cochlea

Oval
window

Round
window

Middle ear
Hammer (malleus)
Anvil (incus)
Stirrup (stapes)
Eustachian tube

Figure 2.1 The outer, middle and inner parts of the ear
Reproduced by kind permission of the Ear Institute, University College London

The eardrum is attached to a tiny bone, called the hammer, or malleus. The malleus is attached to another bone, the anvil or incus, which in turn is attached to a third bone, the stirrup or stapes. These three bones are collectively known as the ossicles and conduct sound vibrations from the tympanic membrane. The ossicles are sited in a small air-filled chamber that obtains its air via a tube called the Eustachian tube that opens at the back of the nose.

Two of the ossicles, the malleus and stapes, are attached to tiny muscles, the tensor tympani and stapedius respectively. These muscles are occasionally associated with specific forms of tinnitus and may also give rise to a sensation of fullness or blockage in the ears (see page 32).

The air-filled space, the three ossicles and the two small muscles constitute the *middle ear*.

The smallest of the ossicles, the stapes, conducts sound into the *inner ear*. This part of the ear is subdivided into the cochlea, which deals with hearing, and the vestibular apparatus, which deals with balance. Sound energy entering the cochlea causes a membrane to vibrate and different parts of this membrane vibrate according to the frequency of the incoming sound. Rows of cells, called hair cells, sit on this membrane. These cells have small rods of muscle protein projecting from their surfaces, which look like hairs under high-powered microscopes and so give the cells their name.

There are two groups of hair cells: inner hair cells and outer hair cells. The vibration of the membrane moves the protein rods of the inner hair cells and this mechanical energy is changed to electrical impulses by the cells. Small nerve fibres underneath the hair cells collect these electrical impulses and convey them to the brain.

Central auditory anatomy

The central auditory system is composed of several structures, some of which have imposing titles such as the inferior colliculus and the medial geniculate body. The names and anatomical descriptions of these structures are not very important in the context of this book. What it is much more important are the functions that the central auditory system performs, which are shown in the form of a flow diagram in Figure 2.2.

The first process is one of recognizing information and making decisions about which sounds must be attended to and which ones can be

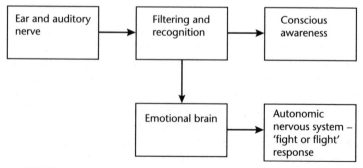

Figure 2.2 The various functional elements of the central auditory system and how they work together

safely ignored. You could consider the auditory brain as having a series of filters, with the purpose of identifying important information and prioritizing it and downgrading unimportant sounds. This is something we all do in everyday life. For example, you can be standing in a busy party with lots of people talking around you, yet if one person mentions your name you will instantly focus in on their conversation. Conversely, you may be so busy doing a task that your friends or family say you are ignoring them or are in a little world of your own.

This ability to either concentrate on sound or block it out is crucial to an understanding of tinnitus. Sound information that is allowed through the filter network is passed to part of the brain called the auditory cortex, which is where we become consciously aware of that sound.

The filtering network can also pass this information to other parts of the brain, particularly the limbic system, which deals with emotions. That is why, if you hear a sudden, unexpected sound, such as a creaking floorboard in the house at night, you may become anxious. The emotional pathways in the brain can, in turn, activate other systems, particularly the sympathetic section of the autonomic nervous system. This is the body's 'fight or flight' response mechanism, the adrenaline centre (see Chapter 8). Thus, not only do you feel anxious but you also become more alert and your pulse starts to quicken, your blood pressure goes up and you breathe slightly faster. If the cause of the creaking floorboard is an intruder, these responses are helpful and may save your life.

This example demonstrates the fact that one of the major functions of your auditory system is to alert you and warn you about danger. Of course, it is not just for that – it also enables sophisticated communica-

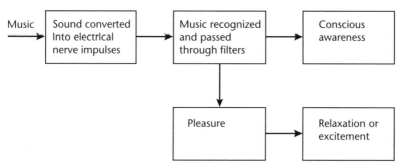

Figure 2.3 How the central auditory system processes sound, enabling us to enjoy music

tion via speech and produces many enjoyable sensations. Figure 2.3 (on the previous page) shows the process that takes place in the auditory system that enables us to enjoy listening to a favourite piece of music.

What the anatomy tells us about how tinnitus develops

To understand how tinnitus develops, we now need to consider research done in the early 1950s by two American researchers, Morris Heller and Moe Bergman.

They placed 80 people who did not have tinnitus, one at a time, in a soundproofed room and told them to listen carefully. They determined that approximately 94 per cent of these people experienced a sound sensation such as hissing, ringing or buzzing when listening hard in silence.

This research was conducted well by the standards of the time, but did attract some subsequent criticism. Interestingly, a recent repeat of the experiment obtained similar results.

Whatever their views on the methodology, the research caused scientists to consider the idea that tinnitus-like sensations are present just below the level of awareness in almost everyone. This is probably due to the healthy, random firing of the auditory nerve at rest or else we could say that it is still busy even when there is no outside sound – it acts 'spontaneously'.

So why do people who do not have tinnitus not normally constantly hear these sounds? Because the filtering network regards them as unimportant and blocks them in a process known as *habituation*. Figure 2.4 shows this random electrical activity being filtered out.

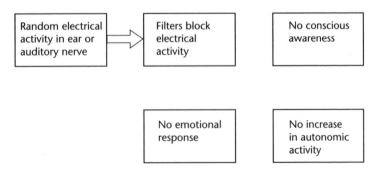

Figure 2.4 The filtering mechanism of the central auditory system working correctly and preventing awareness of random electrical activity

Sometimes this filtering process goes awry and we become briefly aware of a sound sensation. Most people probably experience this for a few seconds at a time. Every now and then, the filtering process can allow the 'spontaneous' neuronal activity through for longer periods. This results in a conscious awareness of sound that can also stimulate the emotional pathways in the brain, which, in turn, can produce an autonomic, fight or flight response (see Figure 2.5).

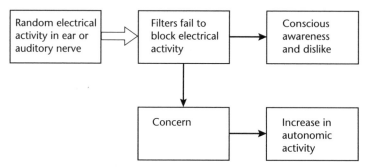

Figure 2.5 The filtering mechanism of the central auditory system can fail and allow random electrical activity to reach other parts of the central auditory system

This increased autonomic activity makes our senses, including our hearing, more acute. Consequently, we notice the spontaneous neuronal activity more. The more we notice the activity, the greater the emotional response to it, resulting in a vicious circle within the central

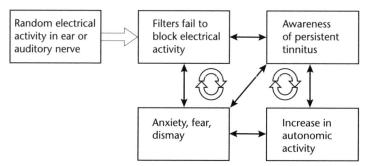

Figure 2.6 The various parts of the central auditory system stimulate other areas, producing positive feedback loops or vicious circles that become synergistic. For example, increased anxiety about sounds causes increased awareness of them and vice versa. The curved arrows show the vicious circles of tinnitus

auditory system. Actually, there are so many interconnections between the various components of the auditory system that the process probably results in the setting up of several vicious circles. If these continue, we become persistently aware of the neuronal activity and tinnitus has arrived (see Figure 2.6, on the previous page).

Once the vicious circles have been set up in the central auditory system, the role of the ear becomes less important. Activation of the emotional pathways in the brain produces the changes in the mood, arousal and thought and behavioural processes that are discussed in Chapter 6.

What causes the filtering mechanism to malfunction?

One possible factor is a hearing loss. This contributes because, as the brain compensates for a hearing loss, it increases sensitivity to sounds that can be heard and, as a consequence, the filters may open wider to allow more information through. Unfortunately, this sometimes allows the spontaneous, random, electrical activity through as well as the important sound information.

Another factor is some kind of emotional shock. Even people whose ears have remained unchanged but have experienced an emotional shock can experience tinnitus as a result. This is because there is increased activity in the emotional brain and this opens the filters. Indeed, many people with tinnitus link the onset of their problem to a life event such as an illness, a bereavement, work or family issues, a car crash or similar.

Finally, there are people who do not seem to have had a hearing change or an emotional upset. It seems that there can be a normal temporary glitch in the filtering mechanism, but, rather than returning to normal, it persists.

Discovering the full picture

It is possible, of course, to experience more than one of these causes – someone with an existing hearing problem may experience an emotional upset, for example, and these two factors together caused the onset of tinnitus.

One helpful tool for understanding the cause of tinnitus is to make a distinction between the *ignition* site of tinnitus, which may be in the inner ear, auditory nerve, emotional brain or other area of the nervous system, and the processes that *promote* the tinnitus into the awareness of the person and *keep* it there.

Tinnitus can be influenced by non-auditory pathways

It used to be assumed that tinnitus was a condition related purely to the auditory system, but, in the early 1990s, some fascinating research was undertaken by Dr Robert Levine, a neurologist working in Boston, USA.

Dr Levine noted that nearly two-thirds of his patients with tinnitus said that it temporarily changed when they made certain movements, such as clenching their teeth, bracing their necks or making a forced smile. In the main, these things increased the intensity of their tinnitus. Furthermore, in people without tinnitus, these movements brought on temporary tinnitus. This phenomenon might be related to the ability that some mammals have to move their ears to help localize sounds, cats being a good example. The brains of these animals have areas that integrate information about the position of their ears and their hearing. Humans have retained this ability, though, as we no longer move our ears in this fashion, the function is vestigial and we do not notice it – that is, until such head and neck muscle movements turn the intensity up, resulting in tinnitus.

More about habituation

As we learned earlier, our brains automatically prioritize the information we receive from our immediate environment, so much of the sensory input coming in does not reach our consciousness. For instance, when you get dressed, your clothing touches your skin, triggering the sensory nerves, which send a myriad nerve impulses to your brain. The brain registers that you have got dressed and then promptly ignores the nerve impulses from the skin. While the clothes are touching the skin, the nerve impulses continue to reach the brain, but you do not continue to pay attention to this information. Regarding sound and hearing, consider a situation where you visit friends who live next to a primary school or a motorway. You might ask them, 'How do you live here with all that noise?' and they will probably reply, 'We don't hear it any more.'

The process by which your brain filters away continuous, background and non-threatening input from your senses, including your auditory system, is known as habituation. This is normal and helpful. In fact, if you were not able to do this, you would be bombarded and bewildered by an array of sensations.

Habituation gives great hope that recovery from troublesome tinnitus is possible as the usual reaction of your body to such sounds is to ignore them. You may find it extremely difficult to believe this, but most people do gradually habituate to their tinnitus. There are two main steps in this process. First, a reduction in agitation, both directly related to tinnitus and any other cause. Second, a change in the meaning of the tinnitus so that, instead of being a sound sensation that the brain gives priority to and must pay attention to, it becomes a background and less meaningful stimulus.

Hyperacusis

As we saw in Chapter 1, hyperacusis is an excessive sensitivity to sound. Other terms for different types of sound sensitivity include phono-phobia, misophonia and recruitment. For a tinnitus and hyperacusis specialist, there are subtle differences between these terms, but, due to considerations of space and usefulness, here we will consider them as a single entity – hyperacusis.

Defining problems associated with sound sensitivity is difficult. We all have a limit to the loudness of sound that we can comfortably tolerate. This limit is not fixed, but varies according to the context of the sound and your mood. Thus, a sound that you can usually tolerate with ease can seem unbearably loud when you are tired, stressed or ill. Similarly, most of us have particular sounds that we dislike, such as chalk screeching down a blackboard or the squeal of a London taxi's brakes.

So, when does a normal reaction to sound change and become hyperacusis? The answer is, when it causes significant distress or even pain to the person who is experiencing it.

How does it develop?

There are probably two main mechanisms by which hyperacusis can develop. First, if the emotional brain is overactive, it can react excessively to sound (see Figure 2.7).

Second, if the auditory system is overactive, it can abnormally enhance sound inputs, which, in turn, causes more activity in the emotional brain and autonomic nervous system (see Figure 2.8). As we have already seen, the emotional brain and subconscious parts of the auditory system are overactive in people with tinnitus, so it is not surprising that hyperacusis is more common in people who have tinnitus than those who do not.

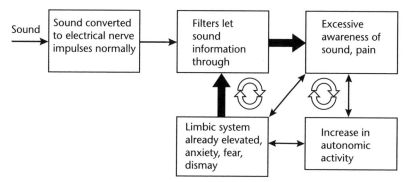

Figure 2.7 Hyperacusis generated by increased activity in the limbic system, causing the filtering network to allow more inputs through to the central auditory system (see the thick black arrows). Vicious circles develop (see curved arrows) – the increased anxiety causes increased auditory awareness, which makes the anxiety worse and so on

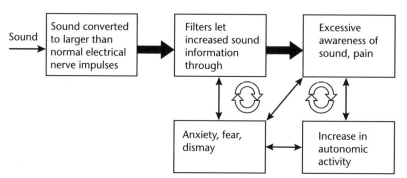

Figure 2.8 Hyperacusis generated by increased activity in the auditory pathways, increasing inputs to the central auditory system to an abnormal level (see the thick black arrows). Vicious circles develop (see curved arrows) – the increased auditory awareness causes increased anxiety, which heightens the awareness and so on

Summary

In this chapter we have presented an overview of what is understood about tinnitus and hyperacusis. This provides you with a framework that enables you to use the information given in the rest of the book, but, if you are interested, we have described some of the mechanisms in more detail in the Appendix.

3

Who has tinnitus and hyperacusis?

Tinnitus

People who develop tinnitus often feel very alone. In fact, this is far from the case as mild tinnitus is extremely widespread and even severe tinnitus is more common than you might think.

Some facts and figures

If we were to ask the general public, 'Have you ever in your life heard a sound inside your head or ears, no matter how mild?' we would receive a large number of positive responses, which may come as a surprise to you. If, however, we asked them, 'Do you presently have a sound inside your head or ears so intense that you are unable to concentrate or sleep?' we would, thankfully, have a much smaller number of yes answers.

The medical literature contains several important studies that have sought to find out how many people have troublesome tinnitus. One of the strongest was a survey of 30,000 adults, led by Professor Adrian Davis, then working for the UK Medical Research Council (MRC) on their National Study of Hearing. The aim was to identify people with what the researchers described as 'prolonged spontaneous tinnitus', rather than those who have noise lasting a few seconds, after exposure to loud noises or in association with a head cold.

Approximately 30 per cent of those questioned had experienced tinnitus at some point in their lives. Ten per cent presently had tinnitus that lasted for more than five minutes; half of them had the tinnitus in both ears, half in just one ear.

The MRC team went on to consider how many of these people had 'severe' tinnitus, the main characteristic of that being a reduction in the ability to sleep. It was found that in 1 in 20 people (5 per cent), their tinnitus was moderately to severely annoying and in 1 in 200 people (0.5 per cent) it was causing a very significant reduction in their quality of life. This last figure equates to over 300,000 of the 61 million people living in the UK.

Another area of interest is how many people seek medical opinion regarding their tinnitus. In the UK, about 7 per cent of adults have consulted their doctor regarding tinnitus, though not all of these were referred to a specialist – in fact, only about a third, representing about 2 per cent of the population.

The medical literature presently available all relates to people in the industrialized, wealthier parts of the world and very little is known about tinnitus in the rest of the world. There are anecdotes, such as tinnitus being seen as a sign of venerable age and maturity in rural China and left-sided tinnitus a sign of divine communication in rural India, but these are notoriously hard to substantiate. The fact that tinnitus has been mentioned for as long as written records exist, however, indicates that it was a problem in societies long before industrialization and, thus, is probably so in non-industrialized societies today.

Tinnitus can affect people of all ages, but is two to three times more common in those over the age of 60 compared to those under 40. The annoyance caused by tinnitus also rises with age. It is interesting to note, however, that annoyance caused by hearing loss increases with age and this becomes progressively more so after 75, while the increase in annoyance with tinnitus is more shallow – a further indication that the link between tinnitus and hearing loss is not as simple as many people assume.

Women are slightly more prone to develop tinnitus than men. Additionally, some women hear more complex tinnitus than men – hearing a cascade of sounds rather than one single tone, for example.

Tinnitus can be heard in one ear, both ears, inside the head or may appear to come from a point outside the body. In those people who hear it just in one ear, there is a clear trend to more left-eared tinnitus than right. Previously this was thought to be due to right-handed people experiencing more noise in their left ear than right (as when you hit a hammer or shoot a gun), but the trend remains even when handedness is accounted for. Sometimes, people initially think that their sound is the central heating or a vehicle idling on the street outside. Once they realize that the heating is off or there is no car, the sound jumps into their ears or head. The simple answer as to why tinnitus is felt to be in a particular place is that the brain is continually making a 'best guess' as to where external sound sources are located and can make mistakes or change its guess and the same is true for the location of tinnitus.

What does tinnitus sound like?

The word tinnitus derives from the Latin verb *tinnire*, 'to ring', and the idea that the experience is 'ringing in the ears' has stuck in the public imagination. In fact, the sound tinnitus can take is almost limitless.

Here are just a few of the descriptions people have given of the sounds and sensations they experience:

- hiss
- sizzle
- buzz
- hum
- engine noise
- grinding
- whispering
- clicking
- music
- white noise
- tone
- whistle
- screaming
- pulsation.

Rather like with the location of tinnitus, the sound probably just represents the brain's best guess. In other words, the brain tries to match the tinnitus to previous sounds that the person has heard, with varying degrees of success. By and large the type of sound that is heard is of no particular significance. There are, however, a few types of tinnitus that we should consider in more detail.

Whispering

Occasionally, it can take the form of whispering or quiet speech. When this happens, it is not uncommon for the affected person, family, friends and even some medical staff to worry that the symptom represents mental illness rather than tinnitus. If the whispering or speech is indistinct and formless, then it can be treated as tinnitus. If, however, clear, meaningful words are heard, then it is a verbal hallucination and needs specialist support from mental health services.

Music

Hearing music in your head is surprisingly common. People may worry that it is a sign of impending mental illness, but, as with whispering, for the overwhelming number of people, this is not the case. It is a normal variant of having a catchy tune stuck in your head all day.

This type of tinnitus is most common in people who have significant hearing loss and it seems likely that the brain is searching for sound information. Unable to locate sound from the outside world, it finds old auditory memories. Hearing aids are normally very effective in controlling this type of tinnitus.

Clicking or pulsation

This is another surprisingly common sound. Sometimes it is caused by a rhythmical contraction of the small muscles in the middle ear (see page 31).

Tinnitus that takes the form of regular pulsation may be caused by blood flow in arteries or veins (see pages 30–1).

Several sounds

Although some people only hear one type of sound, it is common to hear several and, for some people, the tinnitus sound is very complex and changeable. That there is this variation can be a source of burden to some, who long for one, consistent sound rather than the changing, ebbing and flowing sounds they perceive.

Risk factors for tinnitus

There are a number of well-established factors that put a person at an increased risk of developing tinnitus. It is important, however, to recognize that these may not be direct causes of tinnitus, just one factor that can help trigger the problem. A complicating issue is that many of the risk factors are not separate, but linked in some way.

The first and probably most widely known is hearing loss, but the association between tinnitus and hearing loss is by no means simple. It is true that if someone has a hearing loss, he or she is more likely to have tinnitus, but it is also important to note that one-fifth of people who lose all their hearing have no tinnitus and about a third of people with severe tinnitus have otherwise normal hearing. That said, there are many causes and configurations of hearing loss and all seem to increase the risk of tinnitus.

Essentially, there are two ways in which hearing loss may increase the likelihood of tinnitus. First, the cause of the hearing loss may start or ignite the tinnitus. Second, if a person has hearing loss, the external world is quieter, so he or she might be more likely to hear an internal sound that would otherwise be lost among the external sound inputs.

Exposure to loud sound, perhaps at work or in leisure time, over a period of time or as an isolated incident, is associated with a greater risk of tinnitus. Clearly, exposure to loud sound can also lead to hearing loss.

Other risk factors are less obvious. It has been observed that people of lower social class and people who smoke are more prone to troublesome tinnitus than people in other groups. Again, these are not entirely separate factors as it may also be the case that there is an increased likelihood that people of lower social class will work in manual jobs where they will be exposed to noise.

High blood pressure (hypertension) increases the risk of tinnitus, too. This is perhaps due to its effects on the inner ear, though it is important to point out that most people with hypertension do not have tinnitus.

Being anxious or depressed is a risk factor for tinnitus, though it is hard to disentangle the fact that being anxious and perhaps depressed are common responses to tinnitus.

A specific risk factor is that of post-traumatic stress disorder (PTSD). People with PTSD experience disruption in several areas of their lives, with intrusive memories, anxieties and distress that arise from one or more traumatic life events. The involvement of tinnitus in PTSD can be especially disruptive and form a focus for their overwhelming emotions.

It has been noted that many combatants returning from conflicts around the world are experiencing a combination of PTSD, tinnitus and noise-induced hearing loss. Symptoms of PTSD are by no means limited to people who have been involved in war, however. Being caught up in a car crash or witnessing an accident can draw people into the same situation. Having PTSD seems to increase the likelihood of developing tinnitus, but also interferes with people's ability to cope with it.

Childhood tinnitus

Until relatively recently, it was assumed that children do not experience tinnitus. Many researchers, however, had made the mistake of asking children about tinnitus in adult terms and language, in unfriendly surroundings. If care is taken to use the language of children and interview them in surroundings in which they feel relaxed and comfortable, a very different picture emerges.

It seems that about a third of children have experienced tinnitus at some time or other – a figure similar to that for adults. How many children have troublesome prolonged spontaneous tinnitus? The figure is 5 per cent, which, again, is very similar to the incidence in adults, as is the finding that in 1 per cent of children tinnitus can be a severe problem.

It used to be assumed that deaf children do not experience tinnitus.

Once again, this is far from the case. Up to 60 per cent of children born with a hearing impairment report having tinnitus. Of those who are born with normal hearing but subsequently develop a hearing loss – due to infection, injury or other medical factors – the figure is far higher, with some reporting figures as high as 90 per cent.

What is interesting is that many of these deaf children are not troubled by their tinnitus, some perhaps accepting it as normal. It is also interesting to note that most adults with tinnitus do not give a history of childhood tinnitus, which, once more, suggests that children are good at learning to accept and ignore tinnitus.

Hyperacusis

As mentioned earlier, hyperacusis is the symptom of experiencing the world as intensely loud and intrusive. Even low-intensity sound, such as running water, someone turning the page of a newspaper or a mobile phone ringing can be overwhelming and distressing. Many people in this situation withdraw from modern life and are so sceptical that doctors will be sympathetic or able to offer any understanding or therapy that they may not even bother to seek medical advice. As a result, it is difficult to come up with a valid estimate of how many people experience hyperacusis. A study using an Internet survey in Sweden found a prevalence of hyperacusis in nearly 9 per cent of those who responded, but there were factors in the research that mean this is almost certainly an overestimate.

Where we are on firmer ground is to see how many people in a tinnitus clinic also have hyperacusis. There is a consensus that about 40 per cent of people with troublesome tinnitus have some degree of hypersensitivity of hearing and 90 per cent of people referred with hyperacusis have tinnitus. This has led to speculation about links between the two and suggestions that hyperacusis might be an early sign of developing tinnitus or vice versa, but there is little in the way of evidence for these thoughts yet.

One way to calculate the number of people with severe hyperacusis is as follows. If 5 per cent of the adult population have troublesome tinnitus and 40 per cent of these have hyperacusis, a likely and com-monsense figure is that about 2 per cent of the UK adult population have significant hyperacusis.

Even less is known about childhood hyperacusis. What we do know is that children who have a long history of glue ear (where the middle ear fills with viscous sticky fluid) may experience hyperacusis for a while after recovery. Also, children who have had a head injury or are very anxious may be predisposed to hyperacusis. Some children on the autistic spectrum, too, can be hyper-vigilant regarding sounds, finding environmental sounds such as a distant door closing or a phone ringing distracting and intrusive, even upsetting.

Summary

People with tinnitus are very varied – in terms of the causes of their symptoms, in the types of tinnitus they experience and in their reactions. This variability has been a major challenge for tinnitus research. The modern view is that we should consider the physiological mechanisms of tinnitus, the person's reaction to the tinnitus and the beliefs the person develops about the tinnitus if we are to understand the impacts that tinnitus and hyperacusis can have.

4

Medical conditions associated with tinnitus and hyperacusis

We would like to point out that it is easy to read descriptions of medical conditions and imagine that they are affecting you. The conditions we discuss here are, by and large, rare causes of tinnitus and hyperacusis, so do not apply to the great majority of people.

Many people, when they first become aware of their tinnitus, are convinced that it represents some serious underlying problem with their ears and auditory system or even with more general mechanisms within their body. Actually, it is very unusual for this to be the case. The vast majority of people with tinnitus have normal ears and hearing or simply have the normal wear and tear associated with ageing and noise exposure. If you are in any doubt whatsoever, please discuss this matter further with your doctor or an ear, nose and throat specialist.

Having said that, there are a few specific, more commonly occurring medical conditions that are associated with tinnitus and hyperacusis and these are described below.

Earwax

Wax, or cerumen, is produced by the skin of the ear canal as a protective measure.

Many people worry that wax is harmful or theirs is different from other people's. Wax may certainly vary: it may be dry and flaky; soft, sticky or hard; some wax is light in colour; some is dark. These differences, though, are largely genetically predetermined and just represent normal human variation, as do hair or eye colour.

The ear has a way of cleaning itself that involves the eardrum constantly growing new skin cells and these push the older cells to the edge of the eardrum and down the wall of the ear canal. Doctors call this skin migration and it brings wax, dirt and dead skin cells with it. Most ears, left to their own devices, get rid of their wax without the need for syringing or the use of cotton buds.

Tinnitus and hyperacusis are often accompanied by a feeling of ear blockage or fullness, which leads many people to believe that wax is the cause of their problem. This blocked sensation is often a red herring, though, as it is quite unusual for wax to be the cause of these symptoms. Many books and websites list wax as a major cause of tinnitus, but this is rarely the case.

Generally, wax should be left to do its own thing. By all means get your ears checked and, if you're one of those people who regularly develops complete blockage of the ear due to wax, it is, of course, sensible to ask your doctor or an ear, nose and throat (ENT) practitioner to remove it. Wax removal is not something that people can do properly by themselves, though. Doctors see a regular stream of people who have damaged their ears by using cotton buds, matchsticks, ballpoint pens, knitting needles and even hairgrips! Similarly, the use of ear candles to clear wax has been implicated in several cases of significant damage to the ears, so we advise people to seek medical assistance rather than use these devices.

Some people find that having their ears syringed tends to exacerbate their symptoms. If this is the case, ask to be referred to an ENT department as it will be equipped to remove wax by other methods, including the use of special microscopes, suction apparatus and delicate instruments.

Ear infections and glue ear

Many of the people we see in our clinics have been told that their tinnitus was caused by an infection, despite the absence of pain or discharge from the ear. Many received one or more unnecessary courses of antibiotics.

Part of the problem is that people with tinnitus may feel pressure in their ears. This can lead to a misdiagnosis of there being an infection or a problem with the pressure-balancing mechanism of the ear, the Eustachian tube. This results in well-meaning but unhelpful prescriptions of antibiotics or decongestants. Of course, where there is a genuine infection, antibiotics are completely appropriate. We would suggest, however, that someone who is told that their tinnitus is secondary to an infection should be referred to a specialist if one course of antibiotics has not cured the problem.

Otosclerosis

Otosclerosis is an interesting condition in which some of the bone within the ear becomes thicker and develops a spongelike texture. This process prevents the stapes, or stirrup bone, from moving properly and, hence, reduces the amount of sound energy passing from the eardrum to the inner ear, or cochlea.

Otosclerosis is partly due to genetic factors, so, if you have a relative with it, your risk may be increased. There are, however, also other factors at play, such as previous infection with the measles virus or hormonal changes, so women with otosclerosis may observe that their hearing worsens around pregnancy. Whatever the exact cause, the incidence seems to be decreasing and what used to be a common cause of hearing loss in young to middle-aged adults is now quite rare.

Although people with otosclerosis seek medical help because of their hearing loss, the majority will have some tinnitus, which can be intrusive and distressing. Simple examination of the ear and the use of routine hearing tests usually supports a diagnosis of otosclerosis.

Treatment may be simply a question of waiting and retesting, if the symptoms are mild. Hearing aids are often helpful, not only with regard to the hearing itself but also for any accompanying tinnitus. The use of fluoride tablets can help, though in the UK and many other countries this treatment is rarely used.

If these simple measures have not helped, an operation called a stapedectomy or stapedotomy offers the chance of a cure. In this procedure, the surgeon operates down the ear canal, makes a small incision and turns the eardrum forwards to reveal the ossicles or bones of hearing. If the diagnosis of otosclerosis is correct, the stapes will be immobile. The top portion of the bone is removed and a small hole is created with a micro-drill or laser into the inner ear. A prosthetic bone (usually plastic or a mixture of plastic and metal) is inserted and the eardrum is returned to its normal position. Most surgeons insert a dressing in the ear canal that is kept there for a period of several days following the surgery. Somewhere between 80 and 90 per cent of people achieve a dramatic improvement in their hearing following the surgery and similar numbers experience an improvement in or a complete cure for their tinnitus.

We must, however, add a note of caution here. As with any surgery, there are risks attached to this procedure. The main risk is damage to the inner ear. Between 1 and 5 per cent of people find that their hearing is worse after the surgery than before and may even lose their hearing completely. For these reasons, if you have otosclerosis and are contemplating surgery, you need to have a long talk with your surgeon and discuss what his or her outcome figures are. Any surgeon who is regularly performing stapedectomy surgery should be able to tell you what his or her own results are as opposed to the general figures for all ENT surgeons.

Ménière's disease

Ménière's disease is a rare condition that is hugely overdiagnosed. There are many unanswered questions about Ménière's disease and the symptoms vary greatly from person to person. So far as it is possible to generalize, they typically first develop between the ages of 20 and 40. Between attacks, the person initially returns to normal. In a typical attack, a sensation of blockage and tinnitus develops in one ear. Then, after a time, the hearing worsens and the person becomes dizzy, often feeling that everything is spinning around. After a period varying from half an hour to several hours, the dizziness wears off and the other symptoms lessen. The attacks may happen very infrequently or be common.

As the condition progresses over the years, it is common for the person to develop a degree of permanent hearing loss in the affected ear in addition to the episodic fluctuations.

At the onset of Ménière's disease, the most distressing symptom is the dizziness. With time, however, the dizziness often becomes less of a problem and may burn itself out. The tinnitus, by contrast, often becomes more evident later in the course of the condition. This is often a low-frequency sensation, which contrasts with most other types of tinnitus as they tend to be higher-pitched. Also, the disease usually affects only one ear.

The cause of Ménière's disease remains an enigma. It is thought that it is due to a build-up of fluid in the inner ear every so often that temporarily disrupts the hearing and balance organs. The reason for this build-up is not known. In a few rare cases genetic factors seem to be involved.

Treatment usually starts with medication to suppress the dizzy attacks and people are often advised to adopt a low-salt diet. Such measures control the symptoms in the majority of cases. If control is not achieved, surgery may be required. There are currently four techniques that are used.

- *Grommet and pressure device* A grommet is a small, flanged plastic or metal ventilation tube that is inserted into the eardrum under local or general anaesthetic. The grommet provides a connection between the ear canal and the middle ear. When a person feels an attack coming on, they hold a pressure device against the ear. This gently puffs air through the grommet into the middle ear and this is thought to affect the inner ear pressure, thereby preventing the attack.

- *Endolymphatic sac decompression* This is an operation, usually performed under general anaesthetic, in which the bone behind the ear is drilled away until a portion of the inner ear called the endolymphatic sac is exposed. The aim is to remove the bone covering the endolymphatic sac so that the sac can swell more easily and thereby take the pressure off the rest of the inner ear.
- *Vestibular nerve section* This is usually performed under general anaesthetic. A small hole is created in the bone of the skull and a part of the brain is gently lifted out of the way to expose the hearing and balance nerves. The balance nerves are cut, leaving the hearing nerve intact. This is very effective in controlling the episodic dizziness, but does not prevent the hearing from fluctuating.
- *Gentamicin injection* Gentamicin is an antibiotic that is given by injection for serious, potentially life-threatening infections. One of its side effects is that, in high doses, it damages the inner ear, particularly the balance part. This side effect of the drug can be used to control Ménière's disease by selectively destroying the balance function of the inner ear while retaining the hearing function. A small quantity of gentamicin is injected either directly through the eardrum or a previously implanted grommet and diffuses into the inner ear.

All the treatments used for Ménière's disease are designed principally to help with the dizziness. We have a reasonable idea of how they work in this respect, but very little firm evidence for how they help the tinnitus.

Acoustic neuromas

An acoustic neuroma – known as a vestibular schwannoma in medical circles – is a small, benign tumour that grows on the nerve of hearing and balance. This nerve – the vestibulocochlear or eighth cranial nerve – is formed of several different components, some carrying auditory information and some carrying balance information. Acoustic neuromas generally grow on one of the balance nerves, either the superior vestibular nerve or the inferior vestibular nerve.

The vast majority of these tumours grow very slowly, enlarging by less than 1 mm per year, or not at all. As they slowly enlarge, they press against the hearing part of the vestibulocochlear nerve. This eventually results in hearing loss. Tinnitus is a common accompanying symptom and occasionally can be the only symptom. Imbalance or dizziness can also occur.

Apart from a few very rare cases associated with an inherited condition called neurofibromatosis II, the cause of acoustic neuromas remains unknown. The best way to diagnose them, however, is to perform a magnetic resonance imaging (MRI) scan (this and other diagnostic techniques are discussed in Chapter 5).

Because they tend to grow extremely slowly, if at all, many do not need active treatment. Many people with an acoustic neuroma simply undergo regular (often annual) MRI scans to ensure that the tumour remains small. If the tumour is larger when first detected or seems to be a more rapidly growing type, active treatment may be needed. This may be some form of radiotherapy or surgery. Surgical procedures for acoustic neuromas are much safer than they were 50 years ago, but, nevertheless, this is still a major undertaking. Surgery is very effective at removing the tumour, but less effective where tinnitus control is concerned. Approximately two-fifths of people with tinnitus before surgery will get some degree of relief from it after the operation. By contrast, however, about one quarter of those who did not have tinnitus preoperatively will develop it to some degree afterwards.

Sudden sensorineural hearing loss

This is a form of hearing loss that comes on over a matter of hours or a day in comparison to the more usual forms of inner ear hearing loss that develop over years.

Sudden sensorineural hearing loss can be caused by many different conditions, including viral infections of the inner ear, problems with the microcirculation of the inner ear and autoimmune diseases in which the body's defences attack its own tissues. Frequently, however, the true cause remains a mystery.

Because there are so many different possibilities, the clinical course and outcome are difficult or even impossible to predict. Numerous treatments have been tried, including steroids to reduce inflammation and drugs to improve the circulation of the inner ear. There is very little evidence for whether or not any of the treatments have a real effect on accompanying tinnitus. Fortunately, though, many cases of sudden sensorineural hearing loss recover spontaneously.

Pulsatile tinnitus

Although tinnitus may take many forms, most people experience a relatively constant noise, such as whistling, humming or ringing. There are, however, some types that involve rhythmical sounds and these are referred to as pulsatile tinnitus.

The rhythm can be in time with the person's pulse, in which case the tinnitus is likely to be caused by a blood vessel, or unrelated to the pulse, which means muscular causes are likely.

Pulsatile tinnitus is also unusual in that, in some cases, it can be heard by other people, either by putting their ear very close to the affected person or using a stethoscope. This is therefore called objective tinnitus. Pulsatile tinnitus from blood vessels often makes a 'whoosh, whoosh' sound. It can be caused by narrowing of blood vessels or the presence of extra, abnormal blood vessels. It can also be caused by generalized increased blood flow in the general circulation, as seen in some cases of severe anaemia.

Some forms of conductive hearing loss, such as otosclerosis (see above), can also be associated with pulsatile tinnitus. This vascular form of pulsatile tinnitus may have a treatable cause, so, if you think you have this type of tinnitus, do discuss it with your doctor.

When doctors investigate pulsatile tinnitus with scans, X-rays and blood tests, they are more likely to find a definitive cause of it than is the case for other forms of tinnitus. Even so, in most cases the exact cause remains unknown. If the cause is detected, some can be treated and potentially the tinnitus can be cured.

Treatment depends very much on the cause. In the case of anaemia, it can be corrected with medication or a blood transfusion, narrowed arteries can be repaired, abnormal circulations can be removed and conductive hearing losses can be surgically corrected. Unfortunately, however, the majority of people with pulsatile tinnitus do not have one of these easily treatable causes and therefore will need to use the techniques that are described elsewhere in this book.

Pulsatile tinnitus associated with muscular activity is surprisingly common. Many of us experience occasional bouts of this without paying much attention to it. The middle ear – the space between the eardrum and the cochlea – has three small bones, known as ossicles. Two of these small bones, the malleus (hammer) and stapes (stirrup) are attached to small muscles. The function of these muscles is a matter of debate, but is probably to protect us from extremely loud noises. Many people notice that when they are very tired the muscles at the corner of their eye can twitch involuntarily. In a very similar fashion, the muscles in the middle ear can produce involuntary contractions. This can create a sound that people describe as rhythmical popping or cracking. Alternatively, people will experience a sensation rather than a noise and will describe a feeling like having an insect trapped in their ear. This is sometimes known as tensor tympani syndrome. Occasionally, larger muscles in the palate can produce involuntary contractions. In this case, the sound may be loud enough for other people to hear.

It is extremely unusual for there to be a serious underlying cause of these muscular forms of pulsatile tinnitus, so the standard advice for managing tinnitus can help. Nonetheless, it is advisable to discuss this with your doctor.

Snaps and pops

Tinnitus produced by muscular activity or blood flow is sometimes known as a somatosound, or 'body sound'. As well as pulsatile tinnitus (see above), other things that the body does can generate somatosounds. For example, when we yawn or swallow, we open the pressure balancing tube, or Eustachian tube that runs from the back of the nose to the ear, which generates a brief crack or pop in the ear. Generally we ignore this, but some people with tinnitus focus on it and may worry that it is abnormal.

Feelings of blockage are common in tinnitus. If wax, infections or malfunctioning Eustachian tubes are not responsible, what is? Sometimes it is overactivity of the small muscles attached to the middle ear ossicles. We have seen how rhythmical contraction of these muscles can produce pulsatile tinnitus. If the same muscles contract continuously rather than rhythmically, the ear can feel blocked. This is sometimes known as tonic tensor tympani syndrome. An understanding of what is causing this symptom is very helpful and frequently an explanation is the only treatment required.

General illnesses

A common worry among people with tinnitus is that their symptom has been caused by an underlying problem such as hypertension and is a warning that they are about to have a heart attack or stroke. This is almost never true. Indeed, most types of tinnitus are not associated with diseases of the circulation, with the exception of pulsatile tinnitus. Conditions that increase the blood flow around the body, such as severe anaemia or some forms of thyroid disease, can cause or exacerbate pulsatile tinnitus, though, so if you think you have this variant of tinnitus you should discuss the matter with your doctor.

Side effects of drugs

Many people feel that their tinnitus started while they were taking some form of medication. They then, very understandably, see the drug as the cause. It is true that some drugs definitely can cause tinnitus. Certainly, very high doses of aspirin can, though it almost always vanishes as soon as the aspirin is stopped. The dose required to have this effect, though, is many, many times larger than the usual taken for pain or fever. The dosage for stroke and heart attack prevention is even lower than that for pain and so is exceedingly unlikely to cause tinnitus.

Quinine, likewise, can cause temporary tinnitus in very high doses. Such doses are generally only used in the treatment of malaria and are many times greater than the dose used to prevent malaria or treat night-time cramps.

Other drugs that can cause tinnitus include some powerful antibiotics and a few chemotherapy drugs.

The above list of tinnitus-causing drugs is short, yet if we look in a pharmacology textbook we will find that hundreds of drugs have been linked to tinnitus. Why is this? The answer is complicated. Some cases happen by coincidence. For example, having tinnitus is common and having to take blood pressure medication is also common. It is therefore inevitable that some people's tinnitus should start while they are taking such drugs and they link the two. Also, people generally have to take medication because they have developed a problem with their health. Having a health problem is stressful and it is this that starts the tinnitus rather than the medication. Finally, a tiny number of people do seem to have unusual reactions to medication, such that a drug which is safe for almost everyone causes unexpected symptoms in a tiny minority. If you feel that a drug has caused or exacerbated your tinnitus, discuss this with the doctor who prescribed it. In many cases, the doctor will be able to reassure you that the drug is not the cause of the tinnitus. In those rare cases of a drug having had a role in causing the tinnitus, alternative preparations are often available.

People often worry about other chemicals, too. Caffeine is a commonly cited trigger for tinnitus, but there is no real proof of this. Caffeine undoubtedly does have effects on the body and changing the amount of caffeine that you consume can result in symptoms such as a headache. Having a bad headache can, in turn, exacerbate pre-existing tinnitus. We therefore recommend that people with tinnitus should have roughly the same amount of tea, coffee or other caffeine-containing drinks every day.

Some people with tinnitus find that alcohol makes their tinnitus much worse. Some find it has no effect at all. Some find that it improves their tinnitus. This is one of those occasions where a bit of common sense and trial and error is the answer. We must stress that alcohol should always be taken in moderation and, even if you find that alcohol helps your tinnitus, you should be careful not to consume more than the recommended number of units.

5

What therapy is available?

Many people who experience tinnitus feel that they have no one to turn to and there is no real way of treating it. This is far from the truth. While there is no simple pill to cure tinnitus there are many strategies that can help lessen its impact.

One of the first things you can do is find out what services are available in your area. There is no standardized form of tinnitus care and support varies greatly from place to place. Also there is no standardization in terms of the professionals who deliver the care, which can be confusing. Thus, in one city you may have an audiologist looking after you, while in an adjacent city similar care may be administered by hearing therapists or doctors.

People you may meet

General practitioner

In the UK, the first step is to see your doctor, who may refer you to an ear, nose and throat (ENT) or audiology department straight away or suggest that you wait and see if the problem resolves spontaneously. This may seem an odd idea, but, perhaps surprisingly, many cases of tinnitus get better without intervention.

Some GPs can arrange a hearing test at the surgery, using either normal audiometric equipment or a small screening device. They can also treat cases of tinnitus associated with infections or blockage of the ear by wax.

In contrast to many other countries, people in the UK cannot refer themselves to an ENT surgeon or NHS audiology department, but require a letter of referral from their GP.

ENT surgeon or audiovestibular physician

On referral, this hospital-based doctor is likely to be the first person you meet and is usually an ENT surgeon – a doctor who has been trained in disorders of the head and neck and carries out surgical operations. All ENT surgeons have received training in the management of tinnitus, but relatively few regard themselves as tinnitus specialists, though most have a subspecialty interest such as the nose and sinuses, children, tumours of the head and neck or conditions of the ears. The latter group are sometimes known as otologists.

If you have one of the specific medical conditions associated with tinnitus described in Chapter 4, your ENT surgeon may suggest an operation. Otherwise, this is very unusual for people with tinnitus as the vast majority do not need surgery.

In a few areas of the country your GP may be able to refer you to an audiovestibular physician (or audiological physician). These are doctors who have received specialist training in conditions of the auditory and balance system. There are, however, very few audiovestibular physicians in the UK.

Most doctors will take a medical history, examine you and arrange further tests and investigations. Once the diagnosis is clear, most doctors will refer you on to other members of the team for treatment, though a few doctors will want to have a hands-on role in your treatment.

Audiologist

Audiology departments are staffed principally by audiologists – healthcare professionals who are trained to perform tests of hearing and balance. They also fit hearing aids and other devices used in sound therapy. In some tinnitus clinics, audiologists are trained in counselling and a few have some training in psychological treatments, such as cognitive behavioural therapy (CBT). Sometimes the audiologist may be the first professional that you meet after referral rather than an ENT surgeon.

Hearing therapist

In many hospital departments, hearing therapists are the main providers of tinnitus care. These are health professionals who provide a rehabilitative service for people with all types of audiological difficulties. They also undertake tasks such as helping people to use their hearing aids effectively and teaching lip-reading. Unlike audiologists, they do not generally perform hearing tests or fit hearing aids.

In a very few hospitals, doctors can refer people with tinnitus directly to audiologists and/or hearing therapists. The career structure for staff in audiology departments in the UK is currently being reorganized, so their role may alter over the next few years.

Nurse specialist

In a few hospital departments, specially trained nurses will provide your tinnitus therapy.

Relaxation therapist

Relaxation techniques may be supplied by an existing member of the team, such as a hearing therapist, but some services employ specialist relaxation therapists.

Clinical psychologist

Although professional support for tinnitus in the UK is based on an audiological model of tinnitus therapy, a more psychological approach is helpful for many people.

Unfortunately, there is a dearth of clinical psychologists who are also audiologically literate. The clinical psychologists who are available use typical psychological techniques, such as CBT.

Dealing with negative attitudes

As you progress along your tinnitus journey, unfortunately you will encounter many people who have a negative outlook. Unhelpful statements such as, 'tinnitus is untreatable' or 'tinnitus sends you barmy' are all too common.

Even more sadly, some healthcare professionals have these attitudes, too. Not everyone you meet in the healthcare system will be well versed in how to deal with tinnitus. If they say that there is nothing that can be done for tinnitus, what they really mean is that there is nothing *they* can do. The best thing to do is walk away and try to find someone else who *can* help you. Clearly this is not always an easy task, but there are many self-help groups that may be able to steer you in the right direction.

Some people with tinnitus also find that their doctor is reluctant to refer them because he or she subscribes to the 'nothing can be done' point of view. In this circumstance, we suggest that you be polite but persistent. If necessary, see another doctor in the practice.

What to expect from your appointment at a tinnitus clinic

The clinician at the outpatient clinic will ask not only about your tinnitus and hearing but also about your general health, current medications, allergies and employment history. He or she will also examine you. If this reveals that your ears are blocked with wax or the debris from an infection, the doctor may want to examine your ears in more detail under a microscope and carefully remove the blockage.

Hearing tests will be arranged, though in some units these are done before you see the doctor. Most people with tinnitus undergo a hearing test called a pure tone audiogram (PTA). This involves wearing a set of headphones and listening out for very quiet sounds. A PTA is often the only test carried out when investigating tinnitus. You may also have the pressure in your ears checked with a device called a tympanometer, especially if your ears feel blocked or if the eardrums looked unusual when examined. Both the PTA and tympanometry are painless and non-invasive tests.

Further audiometric tests are tinnitus pitch and tinnitus loudness tests. Many people with tinnitus find it surprising that these tests are rarely performed in most tinnitus clinics, but the reason for this is twofold. First, the tests are difficult to perform, which can be frustrating for both you and the tester. Second, and probably more importantly, the outcomes of these tests do not influence the treatment.

During your appointment, you may be asked to fill in one or more questionnaires about your tinnitus and other aspects of your health. Because tinnitus is impossible to measure directly, staff use the scores from the questionnaires to determine the severity of your problem and plan further treatment. Questionnaires are also valuable in assessing your progress. So, try to complete such questionnaires as honestly as possible: it is unhelpful to either overemphasize or minimize your symptoms.

Further investigations that may be required

You may need to go for further tests to check if there are any underlying causes of your tinnitus, particularly if it is only in one ear or if the PTA shows a big difference between your ears. The commonest such test is a magnetic resonance imaging (MRI) scan. This produces detailed pictures of the auditory system, including the hearing nerves and adjacent brain.

MRI scanners use strong magnetic fields and radio frequency energy to produce the pictures. A scan of the auditory nerves takes approximately 15 minutes and involves lying in the machine. Early MRI scanners had very confined interiors and many people felt like they were being put in a torpedo tube, but modern machines are much more open. Also, for an auditory nerve scan, only your head needs to go into the scanner. The machine can still feel slightly claustrophobic, so, if you are worried about this, mention it to your doctor as it may be possible for you to take a mild sedative. Be reassured, too, that the staff are usually very good at putting you at your ease and making you comfortable (see Figure 5.1). Also, an intercom or panic button is available.

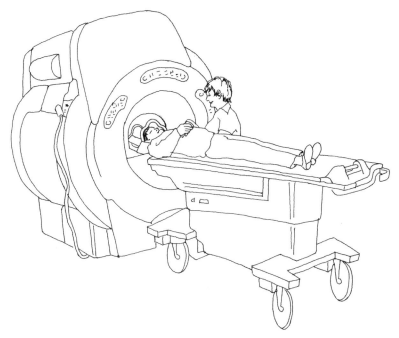

Figure 5.1 A patient undergoing a scan in a modern MRI scanner

MRI scanners are noisy, so it is usual to wear ear defenders for the duration of the scan. Alternatively, sometimes it is possible to listen to music through headphones while the scan is being conducted.

Not everyone can undergo an MRI scan. People with pacemakers or cochlear implants cannot have one due to the strong magnetic field. Those with some types of metallic surgical implants are also unable to have such a scan, though dental implants, dental fillings and ortho-paedic implants, such as artificial joints, do not usually cause problems.

If you need a scan but cannot have MRI or suffer from claustro-phobia, there are alternatives. A computed tomography (CT) scan uses X-rays to produce pictures similar to those produced by MRI. CT scan-ning is much less claustrophobic, much quicker (it usually only takes a matter of seconds) and much quieter than MRI, though the images are slightly less detailed than MRI ones.

If you are one of the few people who cannot be scanned by either MRI or CT, a specialized hearing test called brainstem evoked response audiometry (BSER or ABR) can be used to give more information about the auditory pathways.

Many people undergo these various kinds of investigations, but the number of those who turn out to have a serious problem is very small. In our clinics, for example, approximately 98 per cent of scans are normal. Remember, you don't have a scan because the doctor thinks that something is wrong, but to ensure that everything is normal.

Once the appropriate investigations have been completed, most people can be reassured that they do not have a specific underlying cause for their tinnitus. The small number who do turn out to have a specific medical condition will be likely to have one of the conditions discussed in more detail in Chapter 4.

For most people, the next step is to begin treatment.

What forms of treatment are there?

Reassurance

It may be difficult to believe, but reassurance and explanation are all that many people with tinnitus require. This is because, when tinnitus begins, it is common to be anxious and fearful, but then it usually settles down as the brain gradually acclimatizes to this new sensation as a result of the process of habituation. Also, simply understanding what is causing the problem is a great help in hastening this process.

Neurophysiological model treatments for tinnitus

In 1990, a Polish neuroscientist based in the USA, Pawel Jastreboff, developed a model of tinnitus that stressed that although the ear and auditory pathways in the brain are important in the development and maintenance of tinnitus, other non-auditory pathways are also involved. In particular, Dr Jastreboff noted the role played by the parts of the brain involved with emotion and their interaction with the autonomic nervous system in the body's fight or flight response (see Chapter 8).

Dr Jastreboff, working with an English otologist, Jonathan Hazell, and an English audiologist, Jacqui Sheldrake, created a treatment called tinnitus retraining therapy (TRT). TRT is essentially a mixture of education and counselling about tinnitus, together with sound therapy (see Chapter 10). It is still in use today and there is research to show that it does lessen the impact of tinnitus.

TRT in its original form is quite time-consuming and uses a lot of healthcare resources, so many tinnitus clinics have taken the basic message of the neurophysiological model and applied it in a looser and more flexible fashion. Besides educational counselling and sound therapy, other components such as relaxation techniques are also often added. This approach is called habituation-based therapy and has become the form of tinnitus treatment offered by most UK audiology departments.

Sound therapy

As discussed above, different kinds of sound therapy can be included as part of other therapies, but they can also be used as stand-alone therapies in their own right. See Chapter 10 for more details.

Psychological treatments

It has been known for a long time that tinnitus can cause emotional disturbance and, conversely, emotional disturbance can exacerbate tinnitus. Because of this, various psychological treatments are offered, most commonly cognitive behavioural therapy (CBT).

CBT encourages you to examine how your thought processes may be adversely affecting your behaviour and how to change your ways of thinking with the aim of bringing about improvements. Research has shown that this approach is successful in reducing the impact of tinnitus. As mentioned earlier, however, the big stumbling block is that there are very few CBT therapists who also have a good working knowledge of the auditory system and tinnitus. In the UK, a programme has been set up to teach CBT techniques to audiologists, so things will improve. In the meantime, many CBT techniques are used in other chapters in this book and it is worth giving them a try.

Medication

The use of drugs to treat tinnitus has had a rather chequered history. Many have been tried, but no safe, easy-to-take, effective solution has yet been found.

Tantalizingly, there is one drug that does seem to be able to turn tinnitus off for most people. This is lidocaine, a commonly used local anaesthetic. Indeed, it is regularly used by dentists to numb the gums and teeth prior to dental treatment. Following a lucky accident, it was found that this type of local anaesthetic is able to stop or significantly reduce tinnitus in about two-thirds of people. The effect, however, is very short-lived and it must be administered by intravenous injection, which has potentially serious side effects and can cause cardiac arrhythmias, even death. Many attempts have been made to find a drug that has the lidocaine effect but fewer side effects and can be taken orally. To date this search has been fruitless.

Drugs taken for anxiety and depression are sometimes used for tinnitus and may certainly be useful if you have anxiety and depression in association with the tinnitus, but anxiolytic and antidepressant drugs are only active against the anxiety and depression, not seeming to have any specific action regarding the tinnitus. Of course, sorting out anxiety or depression may ultimately help you to deal better with your tinnitus. If you have any doubt about whether or not you should be taking one of these drugs, discuss it with your doctor or specialist.

It has been suggested that vitamin and mineral supplements can help to alleviate tinnitus. Possibly people with vitamin deficiencies may benefit, but if you do not have such a deficiency and have a normal diet, taking extra vitamins and minerals is unlikely to help and can occasionally even be harmful.

Complementary therapies

Many complementary or alternative therapies have been tried by people with tinnitus, including acupuncture, reflexology, craniosacral therapy and homoeopathy. Few of these therapies have been subjected to rigorous scientific scrutiny. Those that have been were shown to have no specific benefits for tinnitus.

Many of these therapies do produce non-specific feelings of well-being and can certainly help people to relax. This may help you to cope better with your tinnitus, so can be worth a try. If you do, though, be realistic about your expectations and accept that, although you may feel generally better, it is extremely unlikely that these therapies will directly improve your tinnitus. Also, limit the number of therapies that you try (see under Avoiding an endless quest, p. 44) as it can be unhelpful and counterproductive to keep trying multiple treatments.

Novel and experimental therapies

There are often articles in newspapers that herald new miracle cures for tinnitus. These techniques then disappointingly fail to materialize as everyday treatments. One explanation for this is that, quite often when a new form of treatment is tried, it is used with very small numbers of highly selected patients by very enthusiastic doctors and scientists. A wave of enthusiasm can generate apparently good initial outcomes, but, when the technique is applied more widely, it turns out that the initial benefit was a placebo (imagined positive) effect rather than a genuine one.

If your tinnitus is significant, it is possible that you may be asked to participate in a research project investigating a potential treatment for tinnitus. Whether or not you do this is very much a personal choice. People in clinical trials, by and large, receive excellent clinical care and there is always the chance that your tinnitus symptoms will improve. Clearly some trials have attendant risks and you need to make sure that these risks are acceptable to you. As with complementary therapies, it is wise to limit the number of trials you become involved with (see under Avoiding an endless quest, p. 44).

Transcranial magnetic stimulation

TMS or rTMS is an experimental treatment that involves applying strong electromagnetic fields to areas of the brain thought to be involved in the perception of tinnitus. Research has shown some temporary lessening of tinnitus symptoms, but the technique is very much in its infancy and its long-term safety is unproven.

Lasers

Low-powered or soft lasers have been suggested as a potential treatment for tinnitus. Although one or two researchers have claimed success, the overwhelming body of scientific research suggests that lasers are ineffective at controlling tinnitus and can even be harmful.

Drugs

For a long time it was assumed that we had tested all the likely types of medication that might help tinnitus and none was beneficial. Recently, however, our knowledge of the mechanisms that cause and maintain tinnitus has improved. In particular, we are more aware of the role the brain plays. The focus of research has therefore shifted from drugs that act on the ear to drugs that act on the auditory pathways in the brain. Brain chemicals called gamma amino butyric acid (GABA) and glutamate are of particular interest and several pharmaceutical companies are investigating compounds that affect these chemicals. Some research programmes are still addressing drugs that act on the ear, however, such as an experimental drug called AM 101.

Once again, although these trials have been discussed in newspapers and details about them are freely available on the Internet, they are still experimental. It is not yet known whether or not they will have any effect and it is possible that some of the drugs being tried will have significant side effects.

Avoiding an endless quest

Some people create a list of all the possible conventional, complementary and experimental therapies that they can find in books, magazines and on the Internet. They then slowly work their way through this list. This is counterproductive. Every time a new treatment is tried, your hopes will be raised that this is going to be the ultimate solution to your problem. If the treatment does not work, your hopes will be dashed. Furthermore, because one more treatment has been crossed off the list, the tinnitus will seem a little bit worse and a little bit more untreatable than it did before.

If you do still want to try new treatments, it is best to limit yourself to one or two treatments and have realistic expectations about what those treatments might achieve.

6

The impacts of tinnitus and hyperacusis

It is common for people with troublesome tinnitus to argue that those who do not suffer as a result of having it cannot have 'real' tinnitus or at least must have a quieter form or a sound that is easier to listen to. This sounds like common sense, but it is not what the evidence tells us.

The research evidence and clinical experience is that, while people with all types of tinnitus can suffer, equally, people with all types of tinnitus can be OK. If you accept this fact, its liberating implication is that, whatever your tinnitus is like, there *is* a way out and you, too, can be OK.

Having said that, for some people the experience is clearly profound and life-changing. Tinnitus may have become the whole focus of your world and, if you have hyperacusis, that world may have been constrained by external sounds.

When tinnitus and hyperacusis do have an effect on you, it is because a chain of events has been set off. There are four links. You may experience an impact on your:

- thoughts
- level of stress arousal
- mood
- behaviour.

Let us look at each of these aspects in turn.

Impacts on your thoughts

When you are aware of your tinnitus, for the first or fiftieth time, or when there is a change in it, you think about what is happening. The exact content of those thoughts will vary from person to person. Some have calm, neutral thoughts (really!), but some have worrying thoughts. People who are troubled by their tinnitus tend to have thoughts that reflect feelings of despair, persecution, hopelessness, loss of enjoyment, a desire for peace and quiet and beliefs that others do not understand.

Other common themes are resentment about the persistence of the tinnitus, a wish to escape it and, very commonly, worries about health and sanity. There is less research on the thought processes of people with hyperacusis, but clinical experience tells us that they are similar.

Impacts on attention and concentration

If you spend a lot of time thinking about tinnitus or sound, it may be hard to think about other things. Up to 70 per cent of people troubled by their tinnitus talk about having difficulty concentrating. They say that it is hard to read a newspaper or book or follow a TV programme. Some find it hard to focus on conversations and this makes it difficult to socialize. Some people believe that tinnitus will make it impossible for them to focus on their work and will mean they need to take time off.

An important question is whether these difficulties with concentration are due to tinnitus itself or other factors, such as changes in your mood, stress arousal or lack of sleep. There has been very little research in this area and the most likely explanation for these problems is that your powers of concentration are still strong, but locked on to your tinnitus rather than other matters.

Selective attention

As we have seen, tinnitus can become the focus of your world. There is now evidence to show that your attention picks tinnitus as a focus instead of other subjects even if you try hard to prevent it from doing so. The process is partly automatic and partly under your own control.

- The automatic part involves your auditory system giving tinnitus priority over other things that might be going on.
- The part over which you can have more control involves doing things like checking your tinnitus for changes in loudness or quality, comparing it to other sounds (such as a clock, computer, car engine, air conditioning) and checking to see how you are feeling (tired, irritable, anxious) and how you are doing (struggling to read or sleep) or looking for other signs of failure.

Selective attention is an ability that we all have to help us deal with dangers. It keeps us focused when we are faced by a threat. While this is vital to our existence when facing danger, it can become unhelpful when dealing with something like tinnitus. That is what can make tinnitus so intrusive.

This process of selective attention can happen in hyperacusis, too. The focus of your attention is on noise. Again, the process is partly automatic and partly under your own control. You are likely to delib-erately monitor your world for sounds and the automatic part of the process means that you are more likely to detect sounds at ever-quieter levels.

Remember, this process is not inevitable. Many people with tinnitus and hyperacusis concentrate very well on whatever they want. Even if you have been drawn into a process of selective attention, there are ways to relieve the situation, which we will talk about in Part 2.

Impacts on your levels of stress arousal

Physical symptoms of stress

Worrying thoughts inevitably lead to an increase in your level of stress arousal. This can produce physical changes in the body, such as an increase in stress hormones, altered heart rate and increased muscle tension in the body, and these have been the subject of considerable research. If your muscles are sufficiently tense, it can lead to pain, usually experienced as headache or neck or shoulder pain. Other very common symptoms are a churning stomach, nausea, heartburn, an increased urgency and frequency of bowel movements, hot flushes and sweating.

Many people with tinnitus experience pain around the ear or ears. It is also possible for muscle tension to lead to feelings of twitching or fullness in the ear (see Chapter 4).

As stress arousal originates in the brain, many studies have looked to see if tinnitus is associated with changes in the brain. They have found increased activity not only in the areas of the brain concerned with hearing but also in other areas, particularly those concerned with emotion. The conclusion is that suffering as a result of having tinnitus is associated with increased arousal, or neuronal excitability, in several brain areas.

Impacts on sleep

High levels of stress arousal make it difficult to sleep. Sleep disturbance is also one of the most common difficulties experienced by people with tinnitus, so we have devoted a whole chapter to it (see Chapter 11).

Impacts on your mood

Worrying thoughts may lead on to distressing emotions, particularly anxiety and depression.

For many, the changes in mood are not severe, but, for some, these changes are important. One study found that as many as 78 per cent of patients attending a tinnitus clinic could be regarded as depressed in psychiatric terms, though other studies have reported slightly lower figures. Research and clinical experience, however, tell us that the distress experienced is real and meaningful.

While the link between anxiety, depression and tinnitus has been recognized for a long time, recent studies have also pointed to a link between tinnitus and post-traumatic stress disorder (PTSD). It is also clear that hyperacusis leads to high levels of anxiety and depression. For the main symptoms of anxiety and depression, see Table 6.1.

Table 6.1 Common symptoms of depression and anxiety

Common symptoms of depression	Common symptoms of anxiety
• Persistent depressed mood, often worse early in the morning or last thing at night	• Abdominal discomfort
	• Diarrhoea
	• Dry mouth
• A loss of interest	• Rapid heartbeat
• Loss of pleasure	• Muscle tension
• Irritability	• Tightness or pain in the chest
• Restlessness/agitation	• Shortness of breath
• Loss of self-confidence	• Dizziness
• Social withdrawal	• Frequent urination
• Lack of energy/tiredness	• Difficulty swallowing
• Trouble sleeping, especially waking early in the morning	• Sleep disturbance, especially trouble getting to sleep
• Loss of libido	• On edge
• Disturbed appetite – eating too much or too little	• Irritability or anger
• Feeling worthless or guilty	• Concentration problems
• Difficulty making decisions	• Fear of madness or losing control
• Poor concentration	• Feeling detached (derealization)
• Memory problems	• Feeling unreal (depersonalization)
• Thoughts of suicide	

Tinnitus and suicide

Many people troubled by their tinnitus say, 'I would be better off dead' or, 'I would not mind if I was run over by a bus.' They may even complain that they feel 'as if' they could commit suicide. These are, however, usually passive thoughts – that is, they are rarely acted on.

While such complaints should not be ignored, it is extremely rare for people with tinnitus or hyperacusis actually to harm themselves.

From looking carefully at what actually happens to people in tinnitus clinics, we can say that those few people who do commit suicide tend to have been at high risk of suicide even without tinnitus. This subject was researched by Gary Jacobson and Devin McCaslin ('A search for evidence of a direct relationship between tinnitus and suicide', *Journal of the American Academy of Audiology*, 12 (10), pages 493–6, 2001) and they concluded that it is not tinnitus *itself* that leads to suicide, but the accompanying psychiatric conditions serve to amplify the effects of tinnitus for those individuals.

If you have thoughts of harming yourself, it is crucial that you get help from your doctor.

Impacts on your behaviour

If you are troubled by tinnitus the chances are that you have made adjustments to your life to help you cope with it. These tend to fall into recognizable categories.

- *Level of activity* You may have found it a struggle to follow your normal pursuits, so have reduced your level of activity. It is common for people to be concerned that overdoing things will make their tinnitus worse. Alternatively, you may have decided to keep busy to distract yourself – you are 'on the run' from tinnitus, as it were.
- *Using background sound* You may decide always to have some background sound in order to mask your tinnitus. Alternatively, you may make efforts to keep background noises at a very quiet level. The latter is especially true for people with hyperacusis. A difficulty with this is that attempts to limit your exposure to loud sounds can greatly limit what you do.

Impacts on family and friends

Making the kinds of changes described above will almost inevitably affect how you get on with other people. You may find it difficult to be with people and so isolate yourself. Alternatively, you may rely on them much more than before and so avoid being alone.

You may talk about tinnitus more or even all the time, something that friends and family will generally find tiring. Spouses and friends are often at a loss as to how to respond. They may wonder whether asking about tinnitus or listening to complaints about it is being supportive or just focusing attention on it.

If you seek to control the amount of noise the family makes, this will also change how members of the family interact.

For all these reasons, it is common for the changes involved in relation to tinnitus and hyperacusis to place a strain on relationships.

Impacts on work

Some people find that they need to take time off work, usually because of the associated distress or concentration problems rather than the tinnitus itself. Interestingly, in the UK, people are given little credit for tinnitus when seeking social security benefits, but will receive benefits instead for the depression or anxiety that might accompany it.

With work that requires careful listening, such as musicians or sound engineers, people are often reluctant to admit that they have tinnitus in case their colleagues or managers assume they are then incapable of doing their jobs. Even among such professionals, tinnitus itself rarely prevents them from continuing to work in those areas. Indeed, for many people, work of whatever kind is an effective distraction from their tinnitus.

Moving forward

In summary, the impact that tinnitus has on people varies enormously. When it has a significant impact, it is because a chain of events develops. This chain involves changes in thinking, levels of stress arousal, mood and behaviour. The changes that occur can lead to the development of vicious circles that keep distress alive and keep tinnitus at the centre of a person's life.

We shall look at these changes and how to tackle them in more detail in the following chapters and illustrate how you can do this by telling you about two people called Mary and Jim (their names have been changed).

Mary

Mary is in her mid fifties and has had a lot of stress in her life. Her 27-year-old son and his wife are drug addicts. They often have crises, with their health and the police. Over the previous three years, Mary has often had to help them out of these crises and care for their eight-year-old son. Her hobby is gardening, on which she spends a great deal of time, and this had always given her relief from life's stresses.

Mary developed tinnitus while she had an ear infection and it remained after the infection had cleared up. She also has a mild hearing loss for high-frequency sounds.

Mary believed that tinnitus would stop her from finding peace and quiet and she would therefore never be able to recover from life's stresses. She believed that quiet places would allow her tinnitus to become more intrusive and loud sounds would further damage her hearing. She also feared that she would slowly drift into a nervous break-down. See Figure 6.1 for a summary of the process Mary went through. Mary became very anxious and suffered from panic (see Figure 6.2).

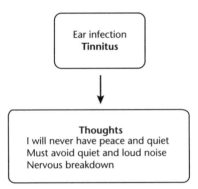

Figure 6.1 Mary's thoughts

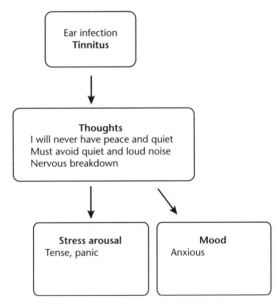

Figure 6.2 Mary's thoughts lead to an increase in her levels of stress arousal and affect her mood

Mary stopped going into her garden because it was too quiet. She made sure that she had some quiet sound around her at all times. She also stopped having her grandson to visit because he was noisy. She gave up doing many of her routine activities and spent a lot of time sitting or lying on her sofa. Often the result of her doing this was that she spent much time ruminating on her problems. These effects on Mary's behaviour are shown in Figure 6.3.

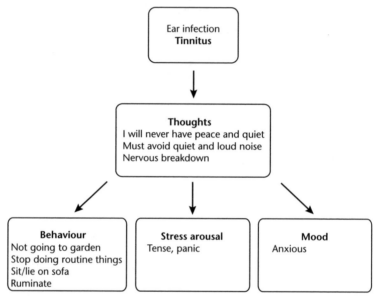

Figure 6.3 Mary's behaviour changes

The general reduction in her activity convinced Mary that she was not doing well and so increased her anxiety. It also meant that she got less out of life, so she began to feel low and found it difficult to get to sleep. She therefore felt like doing even less. Her avoidance of her garden was particularly important. Not having her grandson to visit was also hugely important, with the added sting that she believed she was letting him down. Her low levels of activity gave Mary a lot of time to ruminate on her problems, particularly her tinnitus. Before long, she felt very anxious, despondent and trapped with a head full of tinnitus. Figure 6.4 shows how these areas of Mary's life have become vicious circles that feed each other.

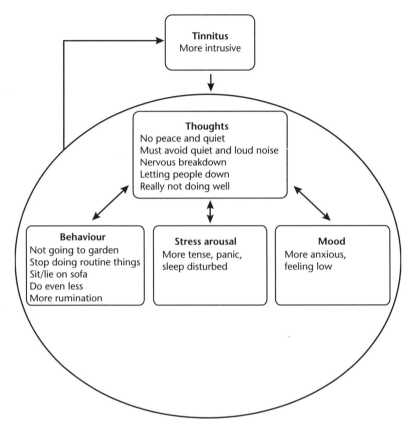

Figure 6.4 The vicious circles have been set up and feed each other

Jim

Jim is in his late thirties and has always worked hard and played hard. He is a successful and inspirational teacher whose work also involves considerable amounts of administration.

Jim's tinnitus emerged one day while he was working on administrative tasks. Audiological investigations and an MRI scan did not reveal any problems and no clear reason was found for his tinnitus. It was said to be 'just one of those things'.

Jim knew that he did not have a serious illness, but he could not see how he could ever function properly or enjoy life again with noise going on in his head. He found it difficult to concentrate on anything other than his tinnitus and especially difficult to focus on the administrative work. The idea that he would not be able to keep on top of his job and his life would be miserable gained a prominent place in his mind (see Figure 6.5).

Jim began to feel incredibly tense and anxious. Not only was he very aware of his tinnitus, but he also started to have headaches (see Figure 6.6).

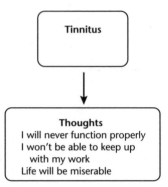

Figure 6.5 Jim's thoughts

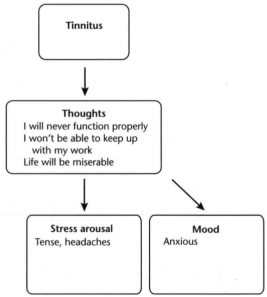

Figure 6.6 Jim's thoughts elevate his levels of stress arousal and affect his mood

Jim refused to 'give in' to his tinnitus. Instead, he worked very hard to keep on top of his job. Because he found it harder to concentrate on the administrative side, he removed all other distractions, particularly noises from his office. He did not think he could produce new, exciting, teaching material for his classes in the way he had always done before. Instead, he 'survived' by rehashing old lessons and, to help him concentrate, insisted on absolute quiet in the classroom. Both he and his students came to dislike his teaching. He also stopped going out with his friends and spent his time at home, trying to catch up on his administrative work. He removed all other distractions and noises there, too. See Figure 6.7 for a summary of where all these changes have left Jim.

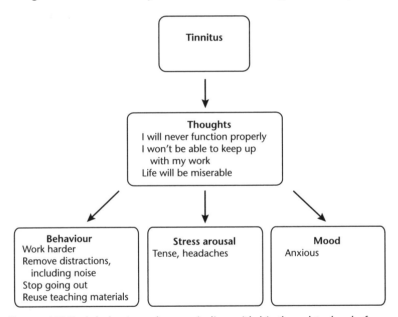

Figure 6.7 Jim's behaviour changes in line with his thoughts, level of stress arousal and mood

The harder Jim tried, the worse things got – he just became more and more tense and got more headaches. The more stressed he became, the more his attention focused on his tinnitus and the more intrusive it became, which made it harder for him to concentrate on his work. He ended up with a 'kettle constantly whistling' in his head and soon he was able to tolerate less and less outside noise. He went on pushing himself to work hard until he became exhausted and totally despondent. Figure 6.8 summarizes Jim's experiences of the vicious circles that got more and more out of control.

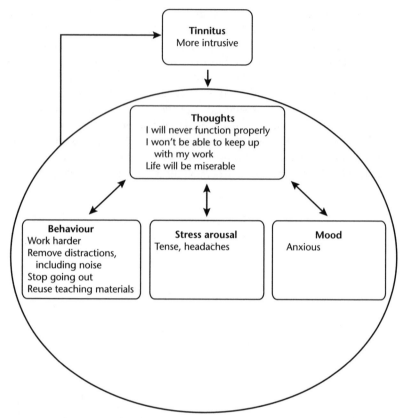

Figure 6.8 Jim is now subject to vicious circles that keep making things worse

This may all seem rather bleak, but we shall see that a detailed under-standing of Mary's and Jim's negative thought processes ultimately pointed the way to how they could deal with their problems and, thus, helped them to return to normal lives.

Part 2
A PROGRAMME FOR RECOVERY

As mentioned earlier, most people are not bothered by their tinnitus and hyperacusis. When they do have an impact, as we touched on in the last chapter, it is because a chain of events is set off. To recap, the links in the chain are:

- a change in how you *think* about things or look at life
- an increase in your level of *stress arousal*
- a drop in your *mood*
- a change in your *behaviour* – what you do and how you lead your life.

Recognizing the different links in the chain is the starting point for your programme of recovery. We shall look at the changes in thinking, levels of stress arousal and behaviour in more detail in the chapters that follow. It is not possible to influence mood directly, but making changes in relation to the other links in the chain can bring about positive changes in mood.

Changes can be achieved by means of CBT, which is described in the following chapters. Sound therapy – one of the most widely used approaches for managing tinnitus – is also discussed, as are sleep problems, which are among the commonest difficulties experienced by people troubled by tinnitus.

7

Understanding and dealing with your thoughts

We have seen earlier in this book how the struggle with tinnitus or hyperacusis comes about primarily because of a series of vicious circles affecting your:

- thoughts
- level of stress arousal
- mood
- behaviour.

The starting point for this chain of events is the impact your symptoms have on your thoughts.

When the tinnitus or external sounds are thought of as threatening, this leads to changes in your levels of stress arousal, mood and in what you do – your behaviour. Your attention also becomes more selective, focusing on the tinnitus or external sounds. Inevitably, this gives you more to worry about.

We know that as your mood gets worse, you are likely to think more about your problems. The way in which you think about things becomes more and more negative. Again, a vicious circle is set up.

We also know that as you worry more about a problem, so the changes in your behaviour become more pronounced. If you think about the tinnitus or external sounds as things that threaten your well-being or even your survival, you will act in the hope of reducing that threat. More often than not, these strategies keep the worrying thoughts alive. For example, avoiding sounds will make your hearing system more sensitive, so that quieter and quieter sounds have an impact on you. This, in turn, can keep you focused on your tinnitus or hyperacusis. In this way, the chain is set up and the vicious circles form, building on each other.

Thinking: the power of thought

Some people suppose that it is impossible to think of their audiological symptoms in anything other than a stressful way. They see them as intrinsically stressful and the distress as inevitable. Remember, however, that the research evidence and clinical experience tells us that things are not that simple. Many people have tinnitus and are OK with it.

The first step on the road to recovery is to recognize that the thoughts you have influence how you feel. We will illustrate this link in the chain with an example that is unrelated to tinnitus or hyperacusis. It is sometimes easier to see this link in events that are less personal to you.

Imagine that you are travelling on a crowded train and, while you are standing, someone pokes you in the back with an umbrella. Imagine this happening a number of times (see Table 7.1).

Table 7.1 What happened on a train journey

What happened
Travelling on a crowded train. Someone poked you in the back with an umbrella – × 2

How would you feel? When asked this, many people say that they would feel annoyed (see Table 7.2).

Table 7.2 How people feel about what happened

What happened	How you feel
Travelling on a crowded train. Someone poked you in the back with an umbrella – × 2	Annoyed

It is important to ask *why* you would feel annoyed (or whatever other emotion you experience). To find out, ask, '*What went through your mind* about the person with the umbrella?' Many people answer this question by saying something like, 'He was being careless' or 'He was doing it deliberately' (see Table 7.3).

Table 7.3 What people think about what happened

What happened	What went through your mind?	How you feel
Travelling on a crowded train. Someone poked you in the back with an umbrella – × 2	He was being inconsiderate or doing it deliberately	Annoyed

If you have a thought like this, feeling annoyed is logical. If, however, you now learn that the person with the umbrella is blind, do you still feel the same? If you feel differently, perhaps even sympathetic, ask yourself again, why? What went through your mind? Maybe it was, 'He is blind so the poke in the back was an accident' (see Table 7.4).

Table 7.4 How new information influences how people think and feel

What happened	What went through your mind?	How you feel
Travelling on a crowded train. Someone poked you in the back with an umbrella – × 2	He was being inconsiderate or doing it deliberately	Annoyed
	He is blind. It was an accident	Sympathetic

The way that you feel (C in Figure 7.1) is associated with how you think (B) about the situation. The situation itself (A) does not determine the emotion (see Figure 7.1).

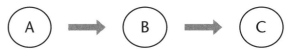

Figure 7.1 The situation (A) leads to a thought about it (B) and how you think about the situation affects how you feel about it (C)

If different thoughts were to be generated by the same situation, then a different emotional state would result (see Figure 7.2).

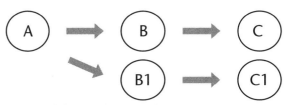

Figure 7.2 Having different thoughts about the same situation can change the way you feel about it

The thoughts that run through your mind and provoke an emotional response are referred to as *automatic thoughts* because they occur without you inviting them.

Of course, we do not think of each new thing as if it is occurring in isolation from other things. Nor do we always think about the same thing in the same way. Instead, how you feel already affects how you think about the next thing that happens. So, if you are feeling stressed, you will think about the event in a stressed way. If you have had a lot of worry recently, for example, you are much more likely to interpret the umbrella in the back as carelessness or even a deliberate act rather than an accident than someone who is in a calm or happy state of mind. In this way, stressed thinking helps to keep you feeling stressed – another vicious circle (see Figure 7.3)!

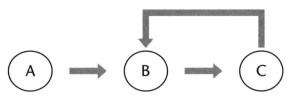

Figure 7.3 Stressed thinking leads to feeling stressed, which leads to more stressed thinking, creating a vicious circle

This feedback process can be very powerful and the type of change that occurs is referred to as *distortion in thinking* or *cognitive distortion*.

Cognitive distortions take place in recognizable ways. For example, there is 'all or none thinking', which is looking at things in absolute black and white categories, or mental filtering, which is when selective attention is paid to negative details.

The effect is something like what happens when you are awake in the middle of the night worrying. Problems seem overwhelming and you believe that you don't have the resources to deal with them. Normally, though they may still exist by lunchtime the next day, they often seem more manageable, but with a distortion in thinking, it is like dropping into 'middle of the night' thinking all the time. The result is that, even though problems are real, you suffer more than you need to.

Such negative automatic thoughts (NATs) have the following qualities. They:

- are uninvited – they just pop up without any effort on your part;
- are plausible – they seem right and may contain a grain of truth;
- have a 'middle of the night worry' quality – they do not fit the facts;

- are unhelpful – they keep you feeling bad and make it difficult to change;
- are involuntary – they can be difficult to switch off.

Tinnitus and hyperacusis can give rise to many different thoughts and, therefore, different emotions. Some people believe their tinnitus to be a natural part of ageing and experience no strong emotions about it. For others, however, thoughts such as, 'This means that I have a serious illness', 'I can't cope with this; I will go mad', or 'It's not fair that I have this', are all likely to lead to distress and this will be made much worse by 'middle of the night' thinking. The result is that their thoughts about tinnitus or external sounds end up being more negative than they need be and they suffer more as a result.

In addition to your current automatic thoughts, your emotions are influenced by your history. Our life experiences, particularly in child-hood, lead us to hold certain assumptions about the world and our place within it. You will have formed some very deep (core) beliefs about yourself and the world. Although you may not be so aware of these deeper beliefs and assumptions, they influence your current auto-matic thoughts and how you respond to all situations, including your tinnitus. Often people are troubled by tinnitus because they believe that it interferes with their ability to live life by the rules that they have followed so far in their lives. 'Perfectionists', for example, have a tough time with tinnitus because of their deeper beliefs.

We are certainly not saying that you should have happy thoughts about tinnitus or hyperacusis! Instead, we are pointing out that there is a slippery slope into *overly* negative thinking that creates and maintains distress. If you are sceptical about the power of thoughts, ask yourself what would happen if you sat for ten minutes and just worried about your tinnitus. Most people don't have to do this exercise to know the answer.

Many say that they try hard to *not* think about their tinnitus. Unfortunately, this strategy rarely works. Indeed, it can even make things worse. It really is better to recognize the importance of thinking and take a systematic approach to investigating and changing any unhelpful ways of thinking that you may have developed.

Discovering what your automatic thoughts are

The first step towards changing any negative automatic thoughts is to discover any you might have about tinnitus or external sounds – that is, find out what's going through your mind. You can do this by having a discussion with your friends or family or audiologist or else note down what goes through your mind when you're feeling distressed by your symptoms. Table 7.5 is an example of the kind of table you could use to record your NATs on a piece of paper or in a notebook when you are troubled by your symptoms.

1 Write down what is happening to your tinnitus or what is happening with external noises in the first column.
2 Write down how you are feeling in the third column. Your feelings can usually be described using one word – irritated, angry, anxious, panic, for example. Also, rate how strong the distress is out of 100 per cent.
3 Ask yourself what went through your mind about the tinnitus or sound and write your answer in the second column. Again, rate how strongly you believe this thought out of 100 per cent.

Writing NATs down like this is much more helpful than just trying to remember them. We have filled in Table 7.5 to give you an example to start you off, together with some other questions that you could ask yourself and feelings you might have.

Table 7.5 Example of a table you could use to record your NATs about your tinnitus or hyperacusis

What happened	What went through your mind?	How you feel
Tinnitus very intrusive	I can never enjoy life with this noise in my head – rating = 85 per cent	Depressed – 70 per cent
	What went through my mind just before I started to feel bad? What am I worried might happen? What does this mean for me?	Sad, anxious, irritated, low, angry, nervous, for example

We recognize that it can be difficult to 'catch' NATs. It may take you many attempts, but persevere – it is worth it! To help you, we have listed the commonest ones in Table 7.6.

You may be more aware of your mood than your thoughts. Your

mood can be used as a clue to the type of NATs you are having. Different moods are associated with different types of thoughts. Generally:

- an *anxious* mood is triggered by ideas that things are going to go wrong;
- a *depressed* mood is triggered by ideas that things already have gone wrong;
- *anger* is triggered by the idea that someone has broken the rules or done something wrong;
- *guilty* feelings are triggered by the idea that you did something wrong.

Remember, NATs often seem convincing and may contain a grain of truth. Ask yourself what the implication of your NAT is. For example, if the first idea that you write down is, 'This noise is so intrusive', it may seem like a therapeutic dead end, but doesn't have to be. It may be useful to ask, 'What does this mean for me?' The answer may be one that you can respond to in a helpful way, but, if you just get another dead end, keep asking the question until you get a more helpful answer. Here is an example of this process at work.

Table 7.6 Typical NATs about tinnitus

What happened	What went through your mind?	How you feel
Intrusive tinnitus	My quality of life has gone I can't be happy I can't enjoy things It's not normal Life will never be the same again I can't do normal things any more I will always feel like this I'll have a nervous breakdown	Low, depressed
	It will affect my physical health It has affected my brain and my ability to think I will go deaf I will never get any peace and quiet I must avoid loud sounds I must avoid silence	Anxious, nervous, on edge
	It's not fair Other people don't understand	Angry, resentful, irritable

This noise is so intrusive.
What does that mean for you?
It will just be there all evening.
What does that mean for you?
I won't enjoy things.
What does that mean for you?
I have lost all quality of life.

It may be true that your tinnitus is very intrusive at that time. It may also be true that you won't enjoy things tonight. These thoughts alone may not be the result of 'middle of the night' thinking, but, the conclusion that you have lost *all* quality of life certainly is. It takes today's difficulty and generalizes it to the rest of life.

By continuing to ask the question, we have got to the heart of the matter here and the thought that needs to be worked on. This approach to discovering your thoughts is called *laddering*, because you take the thought to a new 'rung' each time.

When you are doing this, it also helps to be as specific as you can. For example, if you are worried that you may have a nervous breakdown, it is worth being very clear what that means for you. Some people suppose that a nervous breakdown means losing your reason or running around screaming and pulling your hair out. For others, it means feeling tense all the time and being unable to function in everyday life. Write down what it means for you. When you have done this, you will have something more concrete to work with.

Identifying 'middle of the night' thinking

Once you have identified your NATs, it is important to consider whether or not they contain any 'middle of the night' thinking.

A starting point is to ask if they fall into any of the following usual categories of 'middle of the night' thinking.

- *'All or none' thinking* Viewing situations as either black or white, with no shades of grey. Examples would be, 'My life is perfect' or 'Tinnitus ruins my life', 'Tinnitus is present' or 'Tinnitus is absent' or 'If I can't go to noisy places, I will have nothing in my life.'
- *Catastrophizing (fortune telling)* Predicting negative outcomes without looking at more likely ones, such as, 'My tinnitus will get worse and drive me mad.'
- *Discounting positive information* Telling yourself positive information doesn't count. An example might be, 'OK, I am all right when I am with people (despite tinnitus), but that doesn't mean I am OK.'
- *Emotional reasoning* Thinking something is true because you feel that

it is, ignoring contradictory information, such as, 'I have coped with lots of things in life, but I find tinnitus so hard to manage I feel I must be weak.'

- *Labelling* Putting a global label on things, ignoring information that suggests a less severe conclusion. Saying, 'My life with tinnitus is a total disaster', for example.
- *Magnification or minimization* Giving credit to negative information but not positive information. Examples might be, 'My tinnitus is really loud a lot of the time, so I know I am not making progress', or, 'I am OK sometimes, but that is just because the tinnitus is quieter, not that I am habituating.'
- *Personalization* Believing that others are behaving negatively because of you such as 'My wife is angry because I am struggling with my tinnitus', rather than considering more likely explanations.
- *'Should' and 'must' statements* Holding fixed ideas about how you and others should behave, seeing it as very bad if these expectations are not met – 'I should be able to cope with tinnitus', or, 'The doctors should be able to cure it', for instance.
- *Mental filter (selective abstraction)* Dwelling on one negative detail instead of looking at the whole picture, saying things such as 'My tinnitus was loud by the end of the evening', 'I enjoyed the evening, but had to leave early', or 'I am not coping.'
- *Mindreading* Thinking that you know what others are thinking and failing to consider more likely conclusions. 'People think I am mad because I have tinnitus', or, 'People think I am a burden because I talk about my tinnitus', would be examples of this.
- *Overgeneralization* Making sweeping negative conclusions that go beyond the actual situation, such as, 'My tinnitus got worse when I was vacuuming. I must have total silence.'
- *Tunnel vision* Seeing only the negative aspect of a situation – 'My tinnitus is an unmitigated disaster – it is awful, I can't cope, no one helps, it will never get better', for example.

Make the link between your thoughts and feelings

Once you have identified your NATs, it's helpful to make the link between them and your mood or feelings. For example, the thought 'Life will never be the same again', is likely to trigger a depressed mood. Similarly, the thought 'Tinnitus will lead me to have a nervous breakdown', could trigger an anxious mood. Understanding that NATs trigger moods can help you to change things. Just saying, 'I feel down and I don't know why', is unlikely to help you change.

Also, ask yourself, 'What effects have the thoughts had on my level of stress arousal?' Then, 'How have I changed my behaviour as a result of these thoughts?' The answers to these questions should help you to gain a sense of whether your thoughts are helpful or unhelpful.

Changing your automatic thoughts

Observing your NATs

Take time to observe your thoughts in a very deliberate way. Sit comfortably and just imagine your thoughts passing in front of you like the credits at the end of a film or clouds passing across the sky.

Watch each thought slowly move past and out of sight. Then look for the next one and watch it pass by. Do not resist the thoughts or try to change them, simply observe them. Notice how they come and go.

After a few minutes of this, return to your normal life.

This exercise can help you become less caught up in your thoughts. Notice how thoughts pass and are replaced by other thoughts. This is true of happy, helpful thoughts as well as negative ones. You may come to see thoughts as 'just thoughts' rather than an absolute reality.

Evaluating your NATs

If you are very distressed, you are almost certainly accepting your NATs as accurate. Even though the thoughts seem compelling, remember that they are ideas rather than facts. Even when these thoughts have some truth, it is likely that they have been distorted by 'middle of the night' thinking and so they need to be tested rather than just believed. There are many ways to test such ideas, but here are some questions that we have found help people.

- What tells you that the thought is true? What evidence supports it?
- Is there anything that tells you it is not true? What evidence do you have against it?
- Is there any other explanation for what is happening?
- If a friend asked you for advice about the same problem, what would you say?
- What would a friend say to you?

Asking these questions will cause you to take account of both positive and negative information. Write it all down. Writing things down makes a difference – it is more helpful than just remembering things. See Table 7.7 for an example of how you might integrate this information into the table we used earlier.

Table 7.7 Questions you can ask yourself to test your NATs

What happened	What went through your mind?	How you feel (rate as percentage)	Useful questions	Balanced view (rate as percentage)
What was happening? What was I doing? Was the tinnitus more intrusive than usual?	What went through my mind when I started to feel bad? What am I worried might happen? If this is true, what does it mean for me?	Sad, anxious, irritated, low, angry, nervous	What tells you that the thought is true? What evidence is there against it? Is there any other explanation for what is happening? What would you say to a friend? What would a friend say to you?	

The questions should also help you to think carefully about the commonest NATs people have about tinnitus and hyperacusis. Some seem to be about abstract things and, at first sight, less easy to investigate than others. Good examples are thoughts such as, 'Why me?' and, 'It's not fair.'

There are different ways to answer such questions. One that can be very effective is to make the idea more concrete. Ask, 'What is not fair about my tinnitus or hyperacusis?' If you answer something like, 'It's not fair because I can't do things or won't enjoy things', you have a much clearer idea that you can work on. The five questions listed above and in Table 7.7 will help you explore such ideas in this way, but you may need to use the laddering technique mentioned earlier (see page 66) to get to the heart of the matter.

It can be difficult to find information that goes against a strongly held idea to answer the second question – 'What evidence is there against it?' – so see if, instead, you can come up with an alternative, more helpful idea to replace it. This may be the opposite of your original idea or a toned down version of it. For example, 'I have lost all quality of life' may become 'I have some quality of life.' Think of as much information as you can that supports the new idea.

The third question – 'Is there any other explanation for what is happening?' – is an important one. Recognize the influence of other events in your life. It is easy to suppose that your audiological symptoms cause all your problems, but having tinnitus or hyperacusis does not give you immunity from other problems. If you blame your symptoms for everything, you will feel worse than you need to about them. Moreover, when you try to solve your problems, you may aim at the wrong target.

Another common thought is, 'I can't conquer my tinnitus, so I am weak.' Again, it is helpful to make this more concrete.

What does being 'weak' mean to you? Many people talk in terms of being unable to push tinnitus out of their mind or feeling anxious or depressed and not up to doing things. If it means something like this to you, ask if feeling anxious or depressed is really the same thing as being weak. If so, it means that huge numbers of people must be regarded as weak because tinnitus is very common. Similarly, at any moment in time, one person in five is suffering from major depression. This includes many people whom we would normally regard as strong. It is worth remembering that if you are enduring the burdens of life even though you are experiencing high levels of distress, this probably means that you are, in fact, strong, just as being brave means you feel afraid, but do the best you can anyway.

The important thing to do when you are testing the accuracy of your NATs is to be curious. Don't just accept them as absolutely true. We are not asking you to just think positively here, but, rather, take *everything* into consideration and be careful how much importance you give to certain types of information. Don't just fall into the trap of believing that the negative information is the only important stuff.

It is helpful, too, if you can be inventive and creative when evaluating your NATs. You will be able to look at many thoughts in this way by thinking carefully about them or discussing them with friends and family or your audiologist.

After you have answered the five questions above, think again about your original NAT. See if you can come up with a more balanced version of the idea. Enter this in the fifth column in Table 7.7 and rate, as a percentage, how strongly you believe the balanced idea, then rate the strength of your mood again.

The result of going through this process carefully may be that you realize life is pretty good. Alternatively, you may find that you have a mix of some tough and some OK stuff. Whatever the case, this is likely to be easier than it was accepting that everything is bad. It will also help you to take advantage of the times when you do feel OK.

In order to make the most of having evaluated some of your thoughts, you will need to change the way you do things – we discuss this in Chapter 9.

Changing your deeper thoughts

As mentioned earlier, your NATS are influenced by your history and core beliefs. Sometimes tinnitus does not sit well with rigidly held beliefs, particularly if they have a negative slant on them. We often hear people say things like, 'I have to make sure that I get things right' or, 'I hate letting people down and I make sure I never do it.' Often what follows is, 'If I work hard all the time I will be OK, but tinnitus makes it really difficult to do this.'

A discussion of such deeper beliefs deserves another book, but suffice to say here that repeatedly identifying your NATs will give you a clue to the content of your deeper beliefs. Look out for the same theme coming up time and again. If you repeatedly soften or change your NATs, you may change the corresponding deeper beliefs for the better.

Let us return now to the two people we met at the end of Chapter 6 – Mary and Jim – and look at some of the NATs that they had.

Mary
Mary's NATs and her evaluations of them are set out in Tables 7.8 and 7.9 (overleaf) in the form of an automatic thoughts diary. You will see that she has been able to consider some of her thoughts from different points of view. This has helped to reduce the strength of those thoughts and makes her feel better.

Mary still needs to change how she does things in order to properly evaluate some of her other thoughts. Until she does this, the power of those thoughts will remain quite strong.

Jim
Like Mary, Jim is able to come up with the answers to some of his NATs by making an effort to step outside of his 'middle of the night' thinking and look carefully at all the information available to him. He, too, has completed a couple of automatic thoughts diary pages, which can be seen in Tables 7.10 and 7.11 on pages 74 and 75.

For some of his other NATs, however, he needs to change how he does things in order to find out whether or not they align with the facts.

Table 7.8 Mary's automatic thoughts diary

What happened	What went through your mind? How strong is this idea?	How you feel (rate as a percentage)	Useful questions	Balanced view (rate as a percentage)
Tinnitus very intrusive	Tinnitus will stop me having peace and quiet I will not recover from life's stresses I'll have a nervous breakdown (defined as will not be able to function, lose my reason, have to go to a mental hospital) Rating for strength of idea = 70 per cent	Anxious – 85 per cent	**For:** Tinnitus is always there and I find it difficult to relax I feel anxious I feel like things are getting on top of me I don't sleep well, I stopped doing some things **Against:** I do feel better sometimes – especially if I am busy or with my partner I still function – I cook and do some housework I still manage some of life's stresses – listen to my son telling me about his problems, meet with grandson's social worker I still have my reason – I think and reason through things a lot! **Other explanations:** I have a lot of worry about my son and grandson It is not all tinnitus **Advice to a friend:** Anxiety and sleep problems happen to everyone Ask others for support	Tinnitus troubles me a lot of the time, but not *all* the time I am anxious about a lot of things, but this is *not* the same as having a nervous breakdown or losing my mind I *do* get over life's stresses enough to carry on and some of life is OK Rating for strength of new ideas = 60 per cent Less anxious – 50 per cent

Table 7.9 Mary's automatic thoughts diary continued

What happened	What went through your mind? How strong is this idea?	How you feel (rate as a percentage)	Useful questions	Balanced view (rate as a percentage)
Partner has TV turned up loud	It's too noisy and will make my tinnitus worse I must get away Noise will damage my ears I can't tolerate it I can't have my grandson to stay I am letting him down Rating for strength of idea = 70 per cent	Agitated – 90 per cent	**For:** When there is noise, my tinnitus gets worse and I have to get away from it **Against:** My audiologist told me noise is OK, but I always avoid noise **Other explanations:** It might be anxiety rather than just noise that sets my tinnitus off **Advice to a friend:** Try to be in noise if you can	It might not be just noise – anxiety probably does play a role in setting my tinnitus off Rating for strength of new ideas = 30 per cent Only slightly less anxious – 80 per cent
Thinking about gardening Tinnitus more intrusive	I can't garden any more I can't tolerate quiet places – if I don't have some background sound, my tinnitus will overwhelm me and I will never escape it Rating for strength of idea = 75 per cent	Anxious and sad – 85 per cent	**For:** Background sound takes the edge off tinnitus It's hard at night when things are quiet I *think* that I would not manage without some sound **Against:** My audiologist said it will be OK, but I always have background sound **Other explanations:** Anxiety about quiet makes me check my tinnitus Background sound is tiring **Advice to a friend:** Maybe you should try to be in quiet if you can	Maybe quiet is not so dangerous Maybe anxiety makes me focus on tinnitus Rating for strength of new ideas = 40 per cent Only slightly less anxious – 80 per cent

Table 7.10 Jim's automatic thoughts diary

What happened	What went through your mind? How strong is this idea?	How you feel (rate as a percentage)	Useful questions	Balanced view (rate as a percentage)
Trying to work, tinnitus intrusive	I can't concentrate I can't function properly I won't be able to stay on top of my job	Anxious – 70 per cent	**For:** My tinnitus gets bad when I try to work hard, especially the administration I am behind on my administration work I am not working on my teaching prep I feel worn out **Against:** I have managed to get the work done, even though some of it was late The feedback from my manager has been good **Other explanations:** Maybe I am getting too stressed about my work Maybe I have been given too much work – most people would find it hard **Advice to a friend:** You are doing well in the circumstances Talk to your boss about the amount of administrative work	I am struggling, but I am managing some of the work I am able to function, even if it is not as well as I want to Rating for strength of new ideas = 55 per cent A bit less anxious – 50 per cent

Table 7.11 Jim's automatic thoughts diary continued

What happened	What went through your mind? How strong is this idea?	How you feel (rate as a percentage)	Useful questions	Balanced view (rate as a percentage)
Students making a noise	I can't stand this noise My ears are sensitive and it's too loud I can't teach with this noise going on The noise is making my tinnitus worse and damaging my ears I must tell the students to stop the noise Rating for strength of idea = 75 per cent	Anxious – 80 per cent	**For:** I always get tense when there is noise and my tinnitus always gets worse I find it hard to work It is well known that noise damages your hearing **Against:** My audiologist told me that everyday noises will make my hearing system stronger, but I don't know if this is true so I now always avoid noise **Other explanations:** My audiologist said avoiding noise is making me more sensitive The noise is not dangerously loud, it's my stress levels that are making me react more to sound My stress is also making my tinnitus more intrusive and making it hard for me to concentrate **Advice to a friend:** Follow your audiologist's advice Try to tolerate more noise	The noise levels are not so bad They will not damage me I have just become sensitive because I have been avoiding sound Rating for strength of new ideas = 30 per cent Only slightly less anxious – 70 per cent

8

Stress arousal and relaxation therapy

We will now outline some of the ways in which stress arousal affects you, how it interacts with tinnitus and how you can reduce it.

Our starting point is the nervous system, which includes the brain, spinal cord and all the nerves that travel to every part of the body and back again.

Stress arousal and its effects on the body

One important division of the nervous system is between the *voluntary nervous system* and the *autonomic nervous system* (ANS), or automatic nervous system.

- The voluntary nervous system is so called because it operates under your control. For example, if you want to make a phone call, you must remember to do so, then a message travels from your brain, down your spinal cord to your arm and hand and you pick up the phone. It happens because you want it to happen and you remember to make it happen.
- In the ANS, things happen without you needing to remember to make them happen. In other words, they happen autonomously or automatically. For example, you do not have to remember to keep your heart beating or to breathe.

The ANS does more than just keep your heart beating, though. It will speed it up if you run for a bus and slow it down as you fall asleep, without you needing to make any conscious decision for any of this to happen. It is a remarkable and powerful system. The ANS keeps your lungs working and allows them to speed up, and slow down, as necessary. It regulates your blood pressure and your temperature. You don't consciously think to get goosebumps and shiver when cold or to sweat when hot; the ANS does this for you. The system automatically governs the level of tension in your muscles, allowing them to contract or extend as you do things, such as walking, writing or making a cup of tea. Your digestive processes are also governed by the ANS, as are many aspects of the skin – galvanic skin resistance, or GSR for short, for example, which is what lie detectors measure. Your ears are also under ANS control. Ordinarily, your ears allow you to locate sound, they help you to balance and work out where you are in space without you needing to make any conscious effort. In fact, most things in the body are controlled automatically.

There are two subdivisions within the ANS that regulate the body in different ways (see Figure 8.1):

- the sympathetic ANS speeds the body up and, in so doing, it uses energy;
- the parasympathetic ANS slows the body down, saving energy.

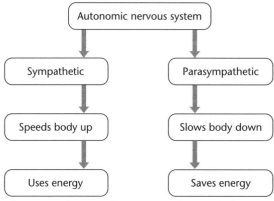

Figure 8.1 The sympathetic and parasympathetic subdivisions of the autonomic nervous system

When the sympathetic part is in operation, the different body functions tend to go faster. Unless you are doing something such as physical exercise, you may notice this in the form of things that are a little out of the ordinary. For example, your heart will beat faster, so you may notice your heart racing or palpitations. The upper part of your digestive system is the exception to this rule – it tends to slow down and, as a consequence, you may get butterflies or feel nauseous.

Table 8.1 lists the common changes associated with increased sympathetic ANS activity. We suggest that you draw up a similar table and use the right-hand column to rate out of ten the extent to which you experience any of these symptoms. You can then repeat this rating process after trying some of the suggestions we make later in this chapter.

The result of increased activity in most bodily symptoms may be a greater feeling of tiredness. Despite this, you may not sleep well because the body needs a lower level of activity if you are to sleep.

Table 8.1 The symptoms of effects of increased sympathetic ANS activity on some of the body's functions and organs

Organ or function	Common symptoms	Your rating (0–10)
Heart	Racing heart, palpitations	
Lungs	Faster breathing, difficulty catching your breath, extra yawning or sighing, giddiness	
Blood pressure	Increases, but apparent only if you measure it	
Temperature	Hot flushes in the trunk of the body, cold extremities	
Digestion	Reduced activity in the upper gut, butterflies, nausea, reflux or heartburn Increased activity in lower gut, increased urgency and frequency of need for the toilet	
Muscle tension	Feeling of tension in the body, pain in any of the major muscle groups – commonly in the head, neck or shoulders, often like a tight band around the head or a thick, muzzy head, and sometimes pain around the ear	
Galvanic skin response	Increased sweating, sticky, clammy feelings, sweaty palms	
Eyes	Slightly blurred vision, more aware of floaters in your vision	
Ears	Feelings of fullness in the ears, pain, more sensitivity to sound, more intrusive tinnitus	

As well as physical symptoms, stress arousal provokes certain psychological changes. In particular, there is an increased focus on whatever is seen as threatening – in this case, tinnitus or external sound. The result is that the tinnitus becomes more intrusive. If you have hyperacusis, you will become more sensitive to external sounds. It can also be harder to pay attention to other things and your memory seems not to work so well. Often, this happens because information about other things is not put securely into your memory stores as your attention is on the tinnitus, external sounds or the consequences of these.

Another common psychological symptom is a feeling of detachment. People describe this in various ways, but often as feeling slightly separate from life, as if you are observing it from a distance or through a glass barrier, rather than actually taking part in it. This is called derealization.

The list of symptoms we have described here is not exhaustive and for some they may not be an important part of their condition. Also, note that some symptoms can come for other reasons, but, if you are worried, talk to your doctor. If you are stressed by tinnitus or hyperacusis, however, it is likely that you will have some symptoms of stress arousal. These are often unpleasant and can be frightening, so it is important to know that when you are experiencing them, your body is not going wrong.

The sympathetic ANS is designed to make the body go faster. An important question is, 'Why have a system that can make you feel so bad?' The answer is that it helped our ancestors survive and it helps us survive.

Imagine a caveman encountering a wild animal. How should he respond? In reality, he has only two options: he either fights the animal or he runs away. Here we have the fight or flight response and it is his sympathetic ANS that puts his body in the right gear to do either.

If he is going to fight, he will need to tense his muscles. The muscles will need to be fuelled. His breathing and heart rate will have to increase to bring oxygen into his body and take carbon dioxide out. One way or another all the physical changes referred to in Table 8.1 will help his body to fight. Interestingly, the story is the same if our caveman decides to run.

Clearly, you are not a caveman or cavewoman! We still have the same ANS, however, and it helps us to deal with today's dangers just as much as it would have helped our caveman, though our threats are more sophisticated, such as muggers, fear of terrorism, financial worries, work stresses or relationship problems. Although these stresses do not necessarily represent threats to our life, they nonetheless provoke the same automatic survival response from the sympathetic ANS.

The problem comes when the threat is one that you cannot literally physically fight or run away from. Tinnitus and hyperacusis are like this. Your body may react to them as if they were wild animals, but you can't physically fight them or run away from them. This means that the energy surge you are given by your sympathetic ANS has nowhere to go and you begin to notice the tense muscles, rapid breathing and heart rate and so on as worrying symptoms. You will naturally say to yourself, 'This is not right; I should not feel like this.'

The vicious circle that then develops, of the symptoms of stress arousal leading to more stress, is all too common. The intrusive tinnitus and increased sensitivity to sound are as much a part of this circle as the increased muscle tension or a racing heart or churning stomach.

Thankfully, help is at hand – from the parasympathetic ANS. You will recall that it slows the body down. The sympathetic and parasympathetic parts of the nervous system work together in a process of reciprocal inhibition. This simply means that one counteracts the other – that is, if you have a lot of sympathetic ANS activity, you will have correspondingly less parasympathetic activity and if you achieve more parasympathetic activity, you will reduce the sympathetic activity.

To do this, you need to deliberately reduce the activity in any one of the body functions referred to in Table 8.1. While most of them are quite difficult to directly manipulate, your level of muscle tension and breathing rate can be changed. Control can be achieved by means of exercises designed to reduce muscle tension and create a more relaxed breathing pattern, such as those described next.

How to help yourself

Stress arousal is a reaction to seeing tinnitus or external sounds as threatening. You will be able to reduce the symptoms of this if you manage to think about tinnitus or external sounds in less threatening terms. Remember, this *can* be achieved, even if it takes time.

While you are working on this, there are things that you can do to reduce the stress arousal reactions you are experiencing. The main way to achieve this is to relax.

Relaxation

There are many very good instructional relaxation CDs or DVDs. There are also some poor ones. If you intend to buy one, look for one that gives instructions for progressive muscle relaxation. Using a CD or DVD has the advantage that you do not have to remember the instructions or keep looking in a book for each next step and the exercises are delivered at the right pace.

That said, we have set out some basic relaxation exercises below to give you some idea of what happens. These will not suit everyone and may need to be adapted for your needs, but they are used widely, and very successfully, in tinnitus and hyperacusis clinics around the world to help people relax properly and stay calm and in control. With practice, they will help you become more aware of tension and be able to relax at the earliest signs of it.

Getting started

Start learning under the best possible conditions to give yourself the best chance of success.

Choose a time to practise when the house is quiet, in a room where you feel at ease. Make sure that you will not be disturbed, so turn off the TV and let someone else answer the phone or the door. Put a 'Do not disturb' sign on the door if necessary!

1 Make sure you are comfortable. Sit in a good armchair or lie on your bed or sofa, making sure that you have some support for your head.
2 Choose a key word – a word that you link with relaxation, such as calm, relaxed, easy, peaceful. You will use this to help induce relaxation below so choose carefully.
3 Create a relaxing picture in your mind. Popular images are a tropical beach scene, a peaceful mountain meadow, being in the woods or a beautiful garden, but you should choose something that works for you. This could be anywhere you have felt relaxed and safe before.
4 Once you have created a visual image, expand on it to include sounds, smells, touch and whatever other information helps to build a really complete image.

Relaxed breathing

Your breathing is controlled by two main muscle groups: the chest muscles and, lower down, the abdominal muscles. Stressed breathing involves quick, shallow breaths and effort from the chest muscles. Relaxed breathing involves slower, deeper breaths, with the breathing out lasting longer than the breathing in. In this kind of breathing, too, the abdominal muscles do more of the work instead. Learning to relax involves learning how to breathe slowly and deeply using your abdominal muscles.

Follow the step-by-step guide below to improve your breathing so it becomes relaxed.

1 Once you have followed the steps under Getting started above, place one hand on your tummy, just below your rib cage. Place your other hand on your chest.

2 Breathe in slowly through your nose into the 'bottom' of your lungs. Send the air down as low as you can. You should feel the hand on your tummy rise. Your chest should move only slightly.

3 When you have taken a full breath in, pause for a moment, then breathe out slowly through your mouth. Be sure to breathe out fully. As you breathe out slowly, the hand on your tummy will lower again. At the same time, say your key word to yourself in your head.

4 Repeat until you have done ten, slow, deep, tummy expanding breaths, each time saying your key word in your head during the out breath. Also, try to make the out breath last longer than the in breath.

Try to keep the rhythm of this breathing smooth and regular, without gulping in a big breath quickly or letting your breath out all at once. It will help to slow down your breathing if you slowly count to three on the in breath (1 . . . 2 . . . 3) and slowly count to four on the out breath (1 . . . 2 . . . 3 . . . 4). Don't forget to pause briefly at the end of each in breath. You should then be breathing like this:

Slow in breath . . . pause . . . slower out breath, repeated ten times.

As you become more practised, you can increase the time you spend on each breath, particularly the out breath. After a little while, you may be able to count to ten on the out breath. If you start to feel lightheaded while practising, though, stop for 15 to 20 seconds, then start again. You may be breathing too quickly.

Muscle relaxation

Exercises to relax the muscles involve tensing and relaxing different muscle groups in the body. If you have rheumatism or problems with your joints or muscles, though, do the exercises very gently. Tensing the muscles makes them slightly tired, which helps them to relax more completely.

Once you have tensed your muscles, hold the tension for a moment and concentrate on that feeling. Then, let go of the tension completely and allow the muscles to relax. Concentrate on how relaxed muscles feel.

As with the breathing exercise, study the sensations that come when you relax. Relaxed muscles feel warm and slightly heavy. Also, pause before you move on to tense the next set of muscles. In this way you will learn the difference between tension and relaxation.

Table 8.2 lists the major muscle groups and gives a brief description of the exercise to do to tense and relax them.

Table 8.2 The muscle groups and relaxation exercises for them

Muscle groups	Muscle relaxation exercise
Hands	Clench fists, feel the tension, hold, then relax and concentrate on the feeling of relaxation in the fingers, hands and lower arms
Upper arms (front)	Bend your elbows, bringing your wrists up to your biceps and feel the tension. Hold a moment, then relax and study the feeling of relaxation in the arms and hands
Upper arms (back)	Raise your arms straight out in front of you – as if sleepwalking. Reach as far as you can with your fingers. Hold, feel the tension on the top of your arms, then relax. Feel the relaxation in your arms
Forehead	Frown or wrinkle your forehead tight. Hold, then relax muscles. See how relaxed your face feels when you let the tensions go
Eyes	Shut your eyes tightly, hold the tension for a moment, then relax. Concentrate on the sensation of relaxation
Jaw	Clench your jaw and bite your teeth together. Feel the tension for a moment. Now relax and focus on how you feel
Tongue	Press your tongue against the roof of your mouth. Feel the tension, then relax
Lips	Purse your lips tightly together. Hold momentarily, relax, then let your lips part slightly
Neck and head	Press your head and neck back into your chair or pillow. Feel the tension. Slowly roll head to the right and feel that tension shift. Slowly roll to the left, then back to the middle. Slowly roll your head forward, touch your chin to your chest. Return to your resting position and relax
Chest	Take a deep breath, fill your lungs with air, then hold for a moment. Slowly release the breath and relax. Breathe in a gentle, relaxed way
Stomach	Pull your stomach muscles in – make your tummy hard. Hold. Now push your stomach out, making your tummy hard again. Pull it in again, then relax

Table 8.2 *(continued)*

Muscle groups	Muscle relaxation exercise
Lower back	Gently arch your lower back and hold the position. Feel the tension. Next, relax and study how it feels
Thighs	Clench your buttocks, press down on your heels, then relax
Calves	Extend your toes away from you, lifting your heels. Hold, then relax
Shins	Lift your toes up and towards you, pushing your heels down. Hold for a moment, then relax
Finishing	When you are relaxed, say your key word or recall your relaxing image and relax even more

Relaxation is a skill and, like any other skill, it needs to be practised. Here are some general guidelines for your practising.

- Develop a routine, practising your relaxed breathing and muscle relaxation every day. It may help you if you find a regular time for each exercise so that relaxation becomes a habit.
- Try not to fall asleep. Once you have mastered relaxation, it can be used to help you get to sleep, but when learning how to relax, it is best to stay awake.
- Record your progress. Draw up a form like that shown in Table 8.3 and make notes each time you have finished practising. As shown in the table, rate your level of tension before and after your practice session. This will help you to monitor how well relaxation is working for you.

Allow yourself time – it usually takes several weeks – to become good at relaxation, but be patient with yourself if you find it hard.

The most commonly heard complaint about relaxation training is, 'I don't have the time to do it.' This can be a real problem, but be careful before settling for this as a reason for not practising relaxation. It may be that the harder it is for you to find the time, the greater is your need to do so. There is also some research that shows when people do reduce their level of stress arousal, they do other things more efficiently. We don't want you to beat yourself up over this, though, so if you can't practise one day, don't give up, just practise again the next day.

Once you have practised tensing and relaxing your muscles for a while, you will be able to relax them without tensing first. This is something you will be able to do anywhere and at any time. In the same way, you can practise relaxed breathing and use your key word or relaxing image to help induce relaxation at any time and in any place. After a while, you may find it helpful to use the two techniques together or one after the other.

Your relaxation record

As mentioned above, Table 8.3 is an example of the kind of form that you can use to keep a record each time you practise your relaxation.

Note whether you practised the relaxed breathing (B) or muscle relaxation (M) exercises. Rate the level of tension you felt before and after each exercise out of ten, with ten being high levels of tension and zero no tension at all. Keeping such a record encourages you to practise and enables you to see your progress and the benefits of relaxation.

Table 8.3 Example of a form to use to keep a record of your relaxation exercises practice

Day/date	Relaxed breathing (B) Muscle relaxation (M)	Tension level before (0–10)	Tension level after (0–10)
Tue 7 June	M	8	4

After ten days or two weeks of relaxation practice, return to your version of Table 8.1 that you made and repeat your rating of the strength of the symptoms that apply to you. This will help to tell you the extent to which relaxation is helping you.

Let us see how Mary and Jim got on when they used these techniques to reduce their levels of stress arousal.

Mary

Mary's NATs that tinnitus would stop her having peace and quiet and ultimately lead to a nervous breakdown led to her experiencing an increase in her levels of stress arousal. This had the effect of making her feel tense and 'panicky'. It also made her sensitive to all sorts of things, including sound.

Mary tried the muscle relaxation exercises and found that she felt calmer while doing them. With daily practice, her tension levels and sense of panic reduced and she felt calmer much more of the time. Also, her reactions to tinnitus and her sensitivity to noise slowly but surely lessened.

Jim

Jim's beliefs that he was unable to function and would not be able to keep on top of his job led to him feeling tense and getting headaches. His levels of stress arousal also contributed to his sensitivity to noise. His belief that noise would damage his ears and worsen his tinnitus, in turn, increased his levels of stress arousal further.

Relaxation played a key part in Jim's recovery. By practising the exercises regularly, the tension he experienced reduced and his headaches eased. The reduction in his levels of stress arousal helped to lessen his selective attention to tinnitus and sound and so set him on the road to habituation. His levels of concentration also slowly improved.

9

Behaviour

The power of behaviour

Your behaviour – what you do in response to tinnitus or external noises – is a vital link in our chain because it has a profound influence on how you understand and think about tinnitus and hyperacusis. That is because, as mentioned earlier, the way you *think* about tinnitus and external sounds, influences your *mood*, your level of *stress arousal* and your *behaviour*, what you do.

The links between thoughts and behaviour

NATs and safety behaviours

Negative automatic thoughts about tinnitus, hyperacusis or, indeed, anything else, usually involve the idea that something will go wrong or has already gone wrong. For example, 'Tinnitus has taken away my enjoyment of life', or 'The restaurant will be loud and I will have noise in my head for days.' Such thoughts involve the idea of danger, which is why they provoke a rise in our levels of stress arousal.

Most people will then try to do something to prevent or avoid the danger. That is, their thinking influences their behaviour. For example, the NAT 'The restaurant will be loud and I will have noise in my head for days' is likely to make you avoid the restaurant. The problem comes when the NAT that drives the behaviour is the result of 'middle of the night' thinking. In these circumstances, your actions to keep safe or solve your problems may stop you from finding out that your worries result from 'middle of the night' thinking. When this happens, your efforts to keep safe are referred to as *safety behaviours* (SBs).

While SBs can reduce your distress in the short term, they do have some important drawbacks. Because they stop you from finding out that your ideas result from 'middle of the night' thinking, they keep your distressing thoughts alive. For example, avoiding noise will stop you from finding out whether you can cope with it or not and reducing the amount you do will reduce the opportunities you have to find out whether you can enjoy life or not.

SBs may even appear to confirm your NATS. For example, if you keep your environment very quiet because you think noise will damage your ears, your hearing may become even more sensitive. It is not the same thing as damage, but it may sound like it to you. Similarly, if you stop doing things because you believe you can't enjoy life any more, life will probably become less enjoyable. There is a fine line between doing things that will help you cope successfully and doing things that amount to SBs.

So, your behaviour can have the effect of keeping your distressing thoughts going or even making them worse. The renewed or strengthened thoughts go on triggering rises in your levels of stress arousal, changes in mood and further changes in your behaviour.

Rumination

Sometimes our thoughts provoke changes in behaviour that, on the face of it, do not seem to be about keeping safe. An important example is dwelling on your tinnitus or hyperacusis so that you think of little else – trying to work out what caused the problem, wondering why the doctors can't fix it or trying to think of your own solutions.

Excessive thinking of this kind is known as rumination. It is rarely helpful. Spending time ruminating reduces your involvement in the rest of life and makes you withdrawn. As a result, you get less out of life, your motivation to do things drops and your mood worsens. All this may affect your relationships with the people you rely on for support. Rumination will also keep your existing NATs going.

Trying to *not* think about tinnitus

Often the reasoning goes something like, 'If I let myself think about it I will feel worse', or 'I might not be able to stop thinking about it.'

This seems like common sense, but trying to *not* think about things can be counterproductive. Pause, sit still and try to not think of an elephant.

What happened? Most people end up thinking of an elephant. The harder they try, the greater the paradoxical effect. That is the way the mind naturally works. This means that doing this will only serve to strengthen your NAT that tinnitus is something that has to be resisted or is exhausting or even something that will overwhelm you.

Changing your behaviour

Changing your behaviour can affect your understanding of what is happening at a number of levels, not just the logical reasoning level. For example, 'I think of my problems all the time, I must be going out of my mind.'

Doing things – as opposed to just thinking about them – provides information from many sources, especially those that are visual, auditory or involve touch and movement. This information is processed in a deeper way than purely verbal information. So, reading about tennis or swimming, say, gives you some valuable information, but practising your serve or a stroke gives you a different and deeper level of understanding. Likewise, the changes that you make to keep safe from tinnitus or external sounds or ruminating about such matters has an effect at many levels and may make you more convinced by your NATs. These changes in behaviour may therefore not only keep your NATs alive but also make them worse.

What should I do?

It is possible that you now feel confused as we have said that both thinking too much and trying to not think of your symptoms are problematic!

What is important here is not only *what* you do but the *consequences* of what you do. So, your behaviour is important if it prevents you from finding out whether or not your worries are as true as you suppose or adds new worries.

The good news is that all this can be turned on its head and changing the way you behave can weaken or disprove existing unhelpful NATs. It can also provide support for more helpful ways of thinking.

How to help yourself

Testing your thoughts and behaviour

First, identify and record your NATs by following the steps set out in Chapter 7.

If you find it difficult to identify your NATs, your behaviour can often give you a clue. Ask yourself what you are doing or have stopped doing because of your tinnitus or hyperacusis. Ask yourself *why* you have made these changes. Your answers should give you clues to your NATs.

The changes people most commonly make with regard to tinnitus are:

- reducing your activity level or giving up activities;
- keeping busy all the time;
- using sound and avoiding silence;
- avoiding everyday loud sounds;
- ruminating on tinnitus;
- trying to not think of tinnitus.

The most important change in behaviour connected with hyperacusis is avoidance of noise. This can take many forms, from using ear plugs when out and about to not going out at all and becoming very withdrawn.

Once you have identified your NATs, the next step is to question them, also using the methods suggested in Chapter 7, which can weaken or even remove many NATs. But some NATs are more resistant. In those cases, you can use the changes you have made to your behaviour to carry out experiments to test your thoughts about tinnitus or hyperacusis. Such 'behavioural experiments' are one of the most powerful ways to bring about change and are a key element in therapy.

There are two main types of behavioural experiment:

1 deliberately do things differently and see what happens;
2 keep things as they are, but carefully observe and collect information relevant to your NATs.

Both types are very helpful, but the exact form your experiments take will depend on what distressing ideas are going through your mind. Let's look at each in turn.

Deliberately change what you do

A commonly held idea, or hypothesis, is that tinnitus will 'take you over' unless you work to push it out of your mind. This can be tested by simply stopping your efforts to resist it.

Allow yourself to think about your tinnitus for a short time and see what happens.

Most people who try this find that their tinnitus does seem a bit more intrusive while they are thinking about it, but then things go back to normal pretty quickly. Their tinnitus does not 'take them over'. In fact, most find that, when they repeat the exercise a few times, they become bored with their tinnitus rather than overwhelmed by it.

Another idea people have is, 'If I don't use sound to take the edge off my tinnitus I will feel much worse.' An experiment to test this might involve spending short periods without your sound generator. Alternatively, if you believe that external sounds will provoke a crisis in you, gradually increasing your exposure to such sounds will help you test this idea. This can be achieved in many ways, such as not using ear plugs in some situations, using an ear-level sound generator or slowly increasing the volume of sounds in your own home before venturing into more noisy situations.

Perhaps you believe that tiredness provokes your tinnitus or that tinnitus makes it impossible to undertake activities, so you greatly reduce the amount you do. Doing less may result in you having less energy and feeling less confidence in your abilities. So, deliberately and carefully increasing the amount you do may give you a different perspective. Many people find that doing more, in fact, reduces their focus on tinnitus and allows them to get more out of life. Doing more activities may also help you to break out of the misery of rumination.

Many people feel that they can cope now, but worry about what will happen if their tinnitus gets worse. It is difficult to test the future, so we have sometimes asked people to deliberately do what might temporarily worsen their symptoms, such as thinking about tinnitus or spending time in a very quiet room.

Usually, they find that these changes don't have as bad an effect as they thought they would or, if they do, they cope well enough. Sometimes they find the changes a bit artificial, but this really does say something about the power of thoughts because, in such cases, doing things has less of an effect than thinking about them.

If you are coping right now, you may want the support of a psychologist, audiologist or hearing therapist before trying changes that might make things worse. It may also be the case that the use of some observational behavioural experiments instead (see below) will help you to recognize that you are coping better than you thought.

Observational experiments

These are helpful when the thought of doing things differently seems too difficult or more information is required before you make bigger changes.

Observational experiments might involve just watching how other people behave or carrying out a survey. For example, if you have the thought, 'It is not normal to have a noise like this in my head', it may be useful to investigate how common tinnitus is (as you are reading this book you will now know that it affects 1 in 10 people in the UK). Collecting information can also be helpful if you have a NAT such as, 'Because of my distress I am letting everyone down', or, 'They think I am weak.' Why not conduct a little survey to find out what your nearest and dearest do actually think. You must, however, be prepared to accept what they say and not find reasons to dismiss it, such as, 'They are just being kind.'

In some observational experiments, keeping a record can be extremely helpful when looking at ideas such as, 'I have lost my quality of life.' Make a diary page with the days of the week across the top and the hours of the day down the left-hand side. This will give you a box for each hour of each day. Write a note about what you do in each box. It can be a headline, such as lunch, work, TV, laundry, play with children and so on. Remember, you are always doing something. If you are just sitting on the sofa thinking, that is what you are doing. If you are standing by the window staring into space, that is what you are doing.

Alongside each entry in your diary, rate how much you enjoyed doing the activity on a scale from zero to ten. As much as possible, fill the diary in as you go along rather than leaving it for hours and trying to remember what you did later.

Keeping this diary for a week or two will tell you a lot about your quality of life. You can also use it to rate how well you managed each activity or what sense of achievement you got from each thing if these are concerns for you. It will also tell you which activities are more helpful to you and which are less helpful and this might help you plan for the future.

This type of diary is called an activity schedule and slight variations on it can be used to find out the reality behind many NATs.

Step-by-step guide to carrying out your own behavioural experiments

The first step is to *plan* it carefully.

- State clearly what the NAT is that you are trying to test.
- Rate how strongly you believe the NAT you are working on as a percentage.
- Try to come up with a possible alternative thought. What might be another way of looking at the situation? What would you say to someone else? Again, rate how strongly you believe this thought as a percentage.
- State what you will do to test out the worrying thought. What exactly will you do? Where? When?
- State clearly what you think will happen if you change the way you do things – that is, what your prediction of the outcome is.
- Make all this as clear and detailed as possible. Be aware of the things you can control and the things you can't that might influence the outcome.

- Work out how you will judge the outcome of your experiment, whether as changes to your tinnitus or sensitivity to sound, your mood, your ability to do other things or something else.
- Write it all down. For an example of a form that you could draw up to record all these aspects of your experiment on, see Table 9.1, which also has examples of the kind of information to enter in each column. Using a form like this will help you to make things specific and fill in any gaps that you might have as you plan it.

Some care is needed when deciding how to measure the outcome. Many people measure it in terms of how intrusive their tinnitus is or how sensitive they are to sound. These may prove helpful, but they do have important drawbacks.

We know that anxiety can make tinnitus worse and it is likely you will feel a little anxious about changing the way you do things anyway. Monitoring your tinnitus and or sound sensitivity will have a similar effect, so be careful what you blame for any increase in the intrusiveness of your tinnitus or sensitivity to sound.

Try combining intrusiveness or sensitivity with a measure of time, such as saying how long it lasts. Alternatively, it may be helpful to

Table 9.1 Example of a form to use to keep a record of your behavioural experiment

The thought (NAT)	The experiment	The prediction	The outcome	Reflection
What thought (NAT) are you testing? Rate how strongly you believe it as a percentage Can you think of an alternative? How strongly do you believe this? Rate as a percentage	What will you do to test this thought? This will probably involve doing something different, but be specific	What do you think will happen when you do the experiment? Be specific	What actually happened? If it was a change in tinnitus or sound sensitivity or mood, how bad was it, how long did it last? How did this match with your prediction?	What have you found out? What does this tell you about the original thought? How strongly do you believe it now? Rate as a percentage How strongly do you believe the alternative thought?

think in terms of your ability to do something, such as watch TV, listen to music, do work tasks, or the extent to which you get a sense of achievement out of doing things or the extent to which you enjoy them. Again, you can rate these things as a percentage. These sorts of measures are usually more helpful than measuring the tinnitus and hyperacusis because they look at the implications of them rather than just the symptoms themselves. Remember, the symptoms are important because of their implications rather than being important in their own right.

Dealing with anxiety

Changing the way you do things is likely to produce at least a little anxiety. Don't make the experiment too easy, though, nor too challenging, otherwise you may not learn much. The level of difficulty should be manageable, but challenging.

If you are facing a very challenging situation, it is best to tackle this in stages, using a series of experiments.

Whatever experiment you decide on, don't just go through the motions – give it your best effort. Also, be careful that you don't subtly avoid situations.

Doing things differently may throw up other NATs. Just asking yourself, 'What is going through my mind just now?' in the middle of an experiment can tell you a lot about what is going on.

When you do things differently, you will be facing your anxieties and this takes courage. Recognize this and be kind to yourself. Understand that your efforts are important. Be aware, if your beliefs about tinnitus or hyperacusis are deeply held, that it may take repeated, stepped experiments to bring about a change to a more helpful state. This might be slow work, but be prepared and keep at it!

Observe what happens

Look closely at what happens when you do things differently. Do this in as much detail as you can. Did your mood change? Did your level of stress arousal change? Did your tinnitus or sound sensitivity change? Did any of these things get better, worse or stay the same? Did you use any safety behaviours or do anything else to protect yourself from your feared outcome that may make you less open to finding things out? Did the experiment have an impact on your thinking?

Reflect on what has happened

Ask yourself what you have learned. In particular, what have you found out about the NAT that you were testing?

This step allows you to compare and contrast what actually happened with the predictions you made in the planning stage. If you do not do this, the experience might be wasted. Taking time to reflect will make the experiences more powerful.

When you have completed the experiment, ask yourself what would have to happen to bring the strength of your NATs and related emotional reactions down further. What could you do to achieve this?

Behavioural experiments are not just about doing things. Planning, observation and reflection are essential components of the process. Changing your behaviour will help you to change your thoughts, which, in turn, will change your levels of stress arousal and mood. When these things change, your tinnitus and hyperacusis will become less intrusive, a more innocuous part of the background.

Let us check in again with Mary and Jim and see how they tested some of their NATs using their own behavioural experiments.

Mary

As we saw earlier, Mary was able to weaken some of her distressing thoughts by asking herself very careful questions about them. For some of her other thoughts, however, she did not have enough information to answer these questions. She could think about the questions and partially answer them so that she had an intellectual answer, but needed to do things differently to gain the experiences that would allow her to know the answers with her heart as well as her head.

See Tables 9.2 and 9.3 (pages 96 and 97) to find out what Mary discovered about herself in the course of her behavioural experiments. Changing how she did things took courage, but it made a real difference to her experience of tinnitus.

Jim

Like Mary, Jim had weakened some of his unhelpful thoughts about tinnitus by carefully questioning them. He too had to do things differently to weaken some of his other unhelpful thoughts. For Jim, this meant doing some things in a way that seemed to run against his instincts to work as hard as he could. Doing less, however, resulted in him having more success.

See Tables 9.4 and 9.5 on pages 98 and 99 for the results of Jim's behavioural experiments.

Table 9.2 Mary's record of her first behavioural experiment

The thought (NAT)	The experiment	The prediction	The outcome	Reflection
NAT = Noise will make my tinnitus worse and it won't get better I can't tolerate the effect of noise Rating for strength of idea = 70 per cent	I will have my grandson Harry to visit for a few hours He is boisterous and noisy I can do this on Saturday morning My husband will be there to help	Harry will make a lot of noise, playing and shouting and will have the TV on loud After 20 minutes of this, my tinnitus will become more intrusive and I will have to escape to my bedroom and let my husband take over I will feel dreadful – a head full of noise, anxious, crying It will take me days to recover and my tinnitus might stay bad for ever	Harry did make some noise He ran in and out of the garden a lot He had the TV on louder than I like it Things were louder than usual, but it was not as bad as I expected I got anxious at the beginning, but this settled down after an hour or so My tinnitus got worse, but only a bit I could cope – I did not go to my bedroom and was able to stick with it My tinnitus was back to normal by the end and I did not have any problems after Harry left My prediction was worse than the reality	Harry's noise was not so bad It did not make my tinnitus any worse I was anxious and that made my tinnitus worse for a bit, but I can tolerate more noise than I thought I can have Harry to visit again and will not feel like I am letting him down My original thought was a form of 'middle of the night' thinking Rating for strength of original NAT = 40 per cent Rating for strength of alternative idea = 60 per cent I need to do it again to be certain
Alternative: Everyday loud sounds will not damage my ears and so will not make my tinnitus worse Any worsening of my tinnitus is temporary and because I get anxious and monitor it Rating for strength of idea = 30 per cent				

Table 9.3 Mary's record of her second behavioural experiment

The thought (NAT)	The experiment	The prediction	The outcome	Reflection
NAT = I can't garden any more The garden is too quiet and will make my tinnitus worse Rating for strength of idea = 75 per cent **Alternative:** The garden is not silent, so I can still achieve something in the garden My tinnitus may be more noticeable, but only because I am worried about it Rating for strength of idea = 40 per cent	I will work in my garden tomorrow afternoon I will spend only 20 minutes there	It will be very quiet and my tinnitus will become much more intrusive I won't be able to concentrate on what I need to do I will feel terrible – anxious and tearful and I will need to get away by going inside and putting the radio on to distract myself I won't be able to distract myself and my tinnitus will remain bad for days	The garden is not completely silent – there are noises, but they are quieter than I have got used to lately I was worried about the impact on my tinnitus and it got a bit worse, but I did manage to do some work I thought I could carry on after 20 minutes and so I actually stayed an hour My anxiety did not get very bad – in fact, I was distracted by all that needs to be done After a while, my tinnitus actually got a bit easier because I was distracted and there were no lasting bad effects	I can tolerate quiet more than I thought It does not make things worse, although worrying about it does make the tinnitus a bit worse Rating for strength of original NAT = 35 per cent Rating for strength of alternative = 65 per cent I need to go back into the garden and try again I will take it slowly This is a relief as maybe my tinnitus has not taken over completely

Table 9.4 Jim's record of his first behavioural experiment

The thought (NAT)	The experiment	The prediction	The outcome	Reflection
NAT = I can't concentrate because of my tinnitus	I will spend less time working	I will fall further behind with work	Knowing that I had to stick at the administration work for only 30 minutes gave me a sense of relief	My original ideas were 'middle of the night' thinking
I must work really hard to keep up with my work	I will do the administration work for only short, set periods (2 x 30 minutes a day) and	I will get more stressed		My tinnitus was capturing all my attention, but this
I am exhausted		My tinnitus will get worse	I found that I worked better and I achieved more by spending less time on	was because I was so anxious
Rating for strength of idea = 75 per cent	will set my alarm clock to tell me when to finish	My headaches will get worse	the job	By spending longer and longer working, I was
		I will feel more despondent	My tinnitus was no worse – maybe even a bit better	just adding to my anxiety and stopping myself from
Alternative: It may be that I am trying too hard and this is making me less efficient and my tinnitus more intrusive Rating for strength of idea = 55 per cent	I will arrange to do other things when the alarm sounds I will not work at home I will do this for a week	The headteacher will complain and I could lose my job	because I knew I would be moving from the task soon I didn't get more stressed I had a sense of having more time for me My predictions of disaster did not come true	getting more positive things out of life Rating for strength of original NAT = 20 per cent Rating for strength of alternative idea = 80 per cent

Table 9.5 Jim's record of his second behavioural experiment

The thought (NAT)	The experiment	The prediction	The outcome	Reflection
NAT = I can't stand noise	I will keep some background sound on in my home for 2 hours a day, using the TV and hi-fi system to achieve this, setting the volume just a tiny bit higher than is comfortable	The low-level sound will make my tinnitus worse and make it difficult for me to concentrate	The initial sound level was low enough for me to tolerate it without anything happening	I thought that keeping noise levels down made sense, but I see now that this was just making my ears more sensitive
My ears are sensitive and everything is too loud		I will feel anxious	Increasing the level very slowly was OK – it allowed my ears to adjust	My anxiety was making me avoid sound and my mind and body were interacting to make life difficult
The noise is making my tinnitus worse and damaging my ears	I will stick with the sound level until I am comfortable with it and keep it at that level for 2 days	The loud sound will make my tinnitus worse and it won't get better	Nothing bad happened	Rating for strength of original NAT = 15 per cent
Rating for strength of idea = 70 per cent		My head will be full of noise	My tinnitus is no worse and, as the days have passed, I have been less worried by sound and my concentration is improving	Rating for strength of alternative idea = 80 per cent
Alternative: Maybe my audiologist is right and sound will make my ears more robust	I will slowly increase the sound level, following the same procedure	Life will be awful		I will repeat this using a radio in my office at work
Rating for strength of idea = 35 per cent				I will work towards allowing a bit more noise in the classroom

10

Sound therapy

Although there is not yet strong evidence regarding the effectiveness of sound therapy, it is one of the most widely used therapies for tinnitus and many people say that they benefit from it.

Reducing contrast

For many people with troublesome tinnitus, it is the starkness of the tinnitus signal that draws their attention to it. By 'starkness' we mean the extent to which it is perceived against the background sound surrounding them. This contrast between the background sound and the tinnitus can be especially strong in very quiet surroundings or if you have a type of hearing loss that means the sounds around you seem very quiet.

Many clinicians try to influence this situation positively using sound so that this contrast is reduced. One of the ways in which they can try to do this is to increase the amount of background sound, which is called *sound enrichment*. In some cases, a hearing aid will increase the awareness of this sound so that the tinnitus is proportionately reduced. Other times listening to an external wideband noise (containing sounds across the frequency range) is beneficial.

These approaches differ considerably from previous attempts to mask tinnitus by listening to intense external sound, the results of which were largely disappointing. Instead, the aspiration is for the chosen sounds to mix in with the tinnitus, so that the starkness of the contrast is reduced and, hopefully, habituation will be more likely.

Stress arousal and its effects on the brain

We have seen earlier the effects that stress and raised alertness can have on the parts of the brain involved in hearing. Sounds can seem louder, more intrusive and more irritating when you are stressed. In fact, because hearing acts as an early warning danger detection system in humans (and other mammals), it would be surprising if there were *not* some link between stress and hearing.

As we have seen, this link is apparent in both tinnitus and hyperacusis. If you are troubled by tinnitus, it is likely that you will feel stressed, agitated and anxious, which causes an increase in how intrusive the tinnitus seems. This leads to greater stress, which, as we saw in Chapter 2, creates the vicious circle of tinnitus.

This explanation is compelling, but scientists are still trying to discover *exactly* what happens in the brain in such situations. There is evidence that the nerve pathways involved in hearing become hyperexcitable. This means that smaller than usual stimuli trigger them into action and they respond more powerfully than they do normally. This certainly helps to explain the major fluctuations in tinnitus that some people experience, sometimes on an hour-by-hour basis. Moreover, as we saw in Chapter 2, it helps to explain how hyperacusis can develop.

Researchers have also suggested that certain neurotransmitters have a key role to play in the experience. *Neurotransmitters* are chemical messengers in the brain and other parts of the nervous system that allow nerve cells to signal to one another.

Research is emerging that indicates they play a role in troublesome tinnitus at the point where the nerve signals leave the cochlear hair cells, activating the nerve of hearing. A neurotransmitter called *glutamate* seems, in some circumstances, to make this signalling process much stronger, perhaps when it is influenced by chemicals released when we are in stressful states.

We mentioned the process of selective attention earlier. This involves an 'executive' part of the brain deciding which sounds to pay attention to and influencing how loud they are perceived to be. A neurotransmitter called *serotonin* has been implicated in this process. Interestingly, serotonin is thought to play a major role in depression, which is often associated with tinnitus.

Research into such mechanisms is urgently under way, as it may be possible to influence them with medication. This might involve infusing a drug into the middle ear in the case of the glutamate or, in the case of serotonin, using a modified version of the Prozac family of antidepressant drugs.

Meanwhile, some clinicians have suggested that sound therapy may help to reduce the excitability of the nerves involved in hearing and tinnitus. The idea is that external sound, when played in an appropriate way, disrupts the way the tinnitus is processed in the brain. It is suggested that it causes the brain to give tinnitus less importance and so the vicious circles are reversed. In hyperacusis, it is suggested that the careful use of sound can lead to the nerves that process sound becoming less sensitive and more robust.

Sound therapy for tinnitus

Sound enrichment

The most informal use of sound therapy is also potentially one of the most useful.

As touched on briefly at the beginning of this chapter, sound enrichment is the tactic of having low-level, pleasant sound around you whenever possible to reduce the starkness of the tinnitus and, in turn, your reaction to it. Over time this may reduce the extent to which the brain seeks out the tinnitus sound.

The sound used is quiet, at a level and of a kind that mixes in with the tinnitus sound but doesn't completely obscure it. Some examples are:

- a fan
- water feature
- quietly spoken radio programmes
- audiobooks
- quiet, uneventful music
- recordings of Gregorian chant and similar relaxing sounds.

One potential danger of using sound enrichment is becoming anxious about times when you will be without it. If you have 'middle of the night' thoughts about being exposed to the tinnitus without this to defend you from it, you might be using sound excessively and this could well prevent you from resolving your anxieties. Extreme examples of this might be carrying a sound source around with you. In this case, professional help may be needed so that you can wean yourself off the sound.

We will return to sound enrichment in Chapter 11 when we discuss using it at night to help with sleep.

Hearing aids for tinnitus

It has long been good clinical practice to offer hearing aids to a person with tinnitus who has associated hearing loss.

As mentioned at the beginning of this chapter, one aim behind this is to increase the stimulation the auditory system in the brain gets from external sounds so that the tinnitus stands out less starkly against it. Another is that, by attending to interesting external sounds, the brain will pay less attention to the tinnitus.

Another reason hearing aids are used is that, if there is hearing loss, this may cause you to strain to hear, which might make you more aware of your tinnitus. Again, it will stand out as the other sounds are more muted in comparison.

How do you know when a hearing aid might be of benefit? Very often, family and friends will remark on a reduced ability to hear, especially regarding catching quick asides and jokes. Hearing when there is background noise may also become a struggle and in some specific situations, such as hearing the checkout person at the supermarket, may be a challenge.

Modern hearing aids are sophisticated and small. Indeed, a single modern hearing aid has more computing power than was used to put Apollo 11 on the Moon! They can be set to meet your own specific hearing thresholds and boost soft sounds, leaving unchanged those sounds that are already loud enough for you to hear. Directional microphones allow the aid to seek out particular sound sources, such as a voice in among background sound.

Systems for the provision of hearing aids vary from country to country. In the UK, the National Health Service provides digital hearing aids free, but they can also be bought from private hearing aid dispensers. The most important aspect to check is, does the person fitting it know anything about tinnitus?

There are recommended guidelines and practices for fitting hearing aids that sometimes need to be amended for tinnitus. An experienced person will know when to do this.

This point is especially important if you are someone who previously would not have thought of having a hearing aid. It is now possible to have one fitted if you have minimal hearing loss, such as an impairment that is limited to a particular frequency range (this is usually the high frequencies). You may even be utterly unaware that you have any hearing loss and, indeed, would not be a candidate for a hearing aid on the basis of hearing loss alone. If this is you, you might well be resistant to this idea, but people in this position who do have a hearing aid fitted often benefit enormously in terms of their tinnitus.

Some people have non-standard hearing loss, such as deafness in one ear, have trouble hearing sounds in the low-frequency range or even hearing that fluctuates on a daily basis. Strategies for each of these situations exist in the hearing aid world and, while not perfect, they offer benefits even in challenging circumstances.

For the most profound types of hearing loss, a cochlear implant can be considered.

The general rule is that better hearing leads to improvements in terms of your tinnitus.

Wearable sound generators

Even though tinnitus maskers, which sought to completely obscure the tinnitus sound using white noise, have gone out of fashion, many people find that wearable sound generators do help them.

Research has indicated that therapeutic sound is likely to be more effective if it is at a quiet level, so that it mingles with the tinnitus rather than masks it, and this is certainly more pleasant than louder sounds.

Devices are now being made that allow an audiologist to customize therapeutic sound to your individual needs using digital technology. This kind of sound therapy is available via specialist tinnitus clinics.

There is a risk, however, that over-reliance on sound can become counterproductive and can even become a form of safety behaviour (see pages 87–8). Portable sound generators are no different in this respect, so it is strongly recommended that, if you do wish to follow this route, you seek advice from a suitably qualified audiologist.

Sound therapy for hyperacusis

The idea that sound can be used to help hyperacusis may seem strange. After all, sound is the very thing that causes the discomfort. If, however, hyperacusis occurs because of hyperactivity in the hearing system, sound can be a useful way to reset the system to its previous levels of activity.

There are several approaches to this. The first is to try and wean yourself off the use of any hearing protection devices you use. These do have a role when using noisy machinery or if you want to go to a loud concert, but, when used in everyday life, they can increase your hypersensitivity even further.

Second, obtain an inexpensive environmental sound generator and quietly introduce the sound of the rain or the ocean into your environment. This can be used overnight, but also while working at a computer or reading. The Hyperacusis Network (see the Resources section at the back of the book) have made some CDs available of pink noise, which is a sound that has all the frequencies present in it, but with the high frequency ones boosted. Some people have helped themselves recover by using these.

Professional help might include the use of ear-level sound generators. While these are available on the Internet, the chances of them being of benefit are significantly higher if they are issued to you by a professional in a framework of understanding about your hyperacusis specifically.

There are two approaches to using such devices. Some clinicians advocate starting at a very low, barely audible intensity, increasing it over time. This is rather like the desensitizing approaches used to treat some other conditions, such as phobias.

Another strategy is to use the device at a consistent and comfortable level, giving the hearing system a reference point so that it can reset or recalibrate itself.

There is little in the way of evidence to distinguish these two approaches in terms of their merits.

One crucial thing to bear in mind with hyperacusis is that you are not at risk of damaging your hearing by exposing yourself to normal levels of sound. While the sounds experienced at a supermarket may be extremely uncomfortable, they will cause you no lasting harm.

Some conclusions

Although sound therapy can be very helpful in the management of tinnitus, it is possible to become overly reliant on it. Also, sound therapy is best carried out under supervision. So, although the advice given in this book is a start, sound therapy is most likely to be effective if you are under the care of an experienced tinnitus practitioner.

11

Sleep

Difficulty sleeping is one of the problems most commonly experienced by people troubled by tinnitus. It has been estimated that 50 per cent of people attending a tinnitus clinic complain of difficulty sleeping. Indeed, for many, sleep problems are the defining feature of their tinnitus.

You may have spotted this chapter in the contents and decided to read it first, but it is best to read the rest of the book before this to help put this chapter in context.

Normal sleep

Many people suppose that a good night's sleep involves eight hours of oblivion, followed by a day feeling refreshed and alert. In reality, a normal night's sleep is more complicated and busier than that.

One important point to note is that there are several stages in a night's sleep. These are divided into two main types:

- rapid eye movement (REM) sleep
- non-rapid eye movement (NREM) sleep.

These different types of sleep are evident in the brainwaves of the sleeping person when examined using an electroencephalogram (EEG).

REM sleep is so called because your eyes twitch. It is also called *paradoxical* or *active* sleep because your physical state is similar to that of someone who is awake, yet you can be difficult to wake up. This type of sleep is closely associated with dreaming.

NREM sleep is divided into stages 1, 2, 3 and 4 – stage 1 is the lightest and stage 4 the deepest sleep.

A normal night's sleep passes through cycles of REM and NREM, each lasting about 90 minutes. You may be interested to learn that we routinely wake in the night as part of this pattern of normal sleep. You may be unaware of these awakenings and just roll over and return to sleep. The first awakening occurs somewhere between an hour-and-a-half and three hours after you went to sleep.

After the first awakening, the periods of REM sleep lengthen and you get less deep sleep for the remainder of the night. Thus, normally, the second half of the night consists of light sleep. This is sometimes experienced as being 'half asleep' and you may even find yourself thinking about things during this type of sleep. The second half of the night also has more awakenings. Again, this is normal.

Our patterns of sleep change with age, so what is normal when you are 5 years old will be different when you are 12 and different again when you are 40 or 70. As you age, you will experience less deep sleep and more awakenings during the night. Young people may wake twice a night, but older adults may wake as often as nine times a night.

Most people get between seven and nine hours of sleep a night, but there are big variations. Some are happy with only four hours, while others prefer ten. Older people tend to sleep less at night, but nap more during the daytime. The amount of sleep also differs from night to night for each of us.

In addition to the different stages of sleep, there is a daily biorhythm, with dips when we may feel sleepy and tend to function poorly (such as in the early hours of the morning and mid to late afternoon). The concept of a siesta nicely allows for these normal dips in arousal.

So, you can see that sleep is complex and a normal night's sleep involves light and deep sleep, dreaming, thinking and waking, as well as periods of stillness. During the day, we also naturally experience different levels of alertness.

Sleep problems

There are various types of sleep problems, but the commonest one is insomnia. This is a delay in getting to sleep at the beginning of the night or getting back to sleep after waking at night.

Almost everyone experiences such troubles at some point in their lives. About 1 in 10 people have persistent sleep problems and this figure can be as high as 1 in 5 in people over the age of 65.

A delay in getting to sleep can be defined as it taking more than 30 minutes to fall asleep. If this happens three or more nights a week and carries on for several months, affecting your daytime functioning, it can be referred to as insomnia.

While it is recognized that sleep is essential, it is not really clear why it is so. A number of possibilities have been suggested and popular ideas include that sleep restores our bodies or conserves energy, although the evidence for such ideas is certainly not complete.

It may surprise you to learn that the evidence for what happens when we sleep poorly is mixed. There is evidence that poor sleep is associated with poorer health. Some researchers, however, have argued that the cause and effect are not clear here as sleep problems often result from poor health or, more probably, from the stress associated with poor health. Poor sleep is certainly associated with stress and other things that go along with stress, such as poor housing, financial and employment problems, even if other health problems are not present.

Other researchers have linked cause and effect differently, arguing that, when people sleep badly, they will feel low or anxious, have poor levels of concentration and notice greater levels of clumsiness and other difficulties in getting through the day.

Some researchers have argued that these problems may result as much, if not more, from the *stress* of poor sleep as from the actual loss of sleep. They would seem to be supported by research studies that have taken the stress out of the sleep loss by paying volunteers to stay awake. The negative effects of sleep deprivation were then not so marked.

The role of stress has also been highlighted by the research finding that over 90 per cent of people who experience insomnia believe that a busy mind plays a more important role in their sleep problems than their physical condition. This seems to be true even when people have important physical symptoms, such as chronic pain. We believe it also to be true of people with tinnitus.

Given that everyone experiences difficulty sleeping at some point, an important question is, why do some people get over it quickly whereas it continues to trouble others? One of the latest and most persuasive ideas is that whatever causes the insomnia in the first place, it is kept going by worry, stress arousal, safety behaviours and inaccurate beliefs about sleep – the same combination that makes tinnitus a problem.

Negative automatic thoughts are a key element in this. Very often, these NATs are about other stresses, usually added to by NATs about the resulting sleep loss. Many of the worrying thoughts are the result of an incorrect understanding of sleep and cause the mind to be very alert, which, in turn, makes sleep difficult. They also lead to a rise in the levels of stress arousal in the body and the effects of this provoke further NATs. It also causes selective attention and monitoring for signs of being awake or of sleep and markers of the effects of poor sleep. People also try to protect themselves from the feared consequences of poor sleep and, often, the changes they make to their behaviour amount to safety behaviours that inadvertently keep the worry alive and keep the mind too busy to sleep. Examples are trying not to think of your problems, keeping the TV on at night and sleeping late in the morning.

What people do during the day can also have an impact on their sleep. For example, taking it easy or napping may stop you finding out if you can actually manage on the amount of sleep you did get. It is also likely to lead to a less stimulating, more boring day that may only increase your feelings of tiredness. These effects can keep your NATs about sleep alive and, in turn, make it harder for you to get a good night's sleep.

Tinnitus and sleep

Remember, most people who have tinnitus are not troubled by it and up to 50 per cent of those who do seek help for their tinnitus sleep well. This tells us that it is possible to have tinnitus *and* sleep well.

The tinnitus of people who sleep badly is not different from that of those who sleep well. They tend to sleep badly because of worry, raised levels of stress arousal, safety behaviours and inaccurate beliefs about sleep, not simply because they have tinnitus. Of course, it may be that worry about the tinnitus starts the sleep problem off.

Bedtime involves a number of changes that can affect your experience of tinnitus. There is usually a change in noise levels as you are likely to turn the TV off, stop talking and, if you wear them, take your hearing aids or sound generators out. When such changes create a stark difference between the background and tinnitus sound, the tinnitus can feel more noticeable.

Bedtime may also be the first time you are free of distractions and your mind has more opportunity to focus on your tinnitus and the cares of the day.

Remember, too, that a normal night's sleep involves several awakenings. If you are anxious about your tinnitus, it may capture your attention when you wake and, if this sets up a chain of NATs, a rise in your levels of stress arousal and changes in behaviour, it may take a long time for you to return to sleep. Again, these changes can make your tinnitus more noticeable.

In each case, it is the environment that changes rather than the tinnitus, but the effect is to make the tinnitus more intrusive.

How to help yourself

Correct any inaccurate beliefs about sleep

Take the time to carefully reflect on your general beliefs about sleep. Perhaps you think that sleep is meant to be a sort of coma state from beginning to end, or you think your sleep is not what it was.

It will help if you recognize it for what it really is – a period of time that involves many changes between deep and light sleep, dreams, maybe even some thinking and certainly several awakenings. Also, people do not necessarily wake feeling refreshed, but are often sleepy and sluggish for some time before being fully awake.

Create an accurate record of your sleep and daytime functioning

When people who sleep badly are asked about their sleep in a clinic, they tend to overestimate how bad the problem is. Objective recordings (EEGs) of people's sleep often indicate that they are getting more sleep than they thought.

It is rarely possible to have such recordings made, however, so a practical and helpful compromise is to keep a sleep diary, such as the example given in Table 11.1. You record how long you spend in bed, how long you take to fall asleep, how much sleep you get, how often you are awake in the night and so on. Have a guess at things such as how long it takes you to fall asleep or how much time you are awake in the night – don't watch the clock. You may be surprised to learn that people's guesses are usually pretty accurate, to within five or ten minutes, which is accurate enough.

Work out how much time you spend in bed by calculating the difference between when you got into bed and when you got up. Take away from this figure all the time you were in bed but awake to calculate the time you spent asleep.

Complete the diary on a daily basis within an hour of getting up. Fill in the column for Monday night's sleep on Tuesday morning, the column for Tuesday on Wednesday morning and so on. At the end of the day, when you can reflect on how things have gone, at the bottom of each column, make a judgement as to how well you functioned during the day. Did you do what you set out to and how well did you do it? This part of the diary is looking at the effects on you of the previous night's sleep.

Keep filling in the diary for two weeks. It will be more accurate and informative than relying on your distressed thoughts about it. Also, if you carry it on, you can use it to judge the benefits of any changes you make. If you like, the information from the diary can be summarized in graphs using a computer program such as Excel.

Table 11.1 Example of a sleep diary

	Example	Monday	Tuesday	Wednesday	Thursday	Friday	Saturday	Sunday
Time spent napping in the day	30 mins							
Amount of medication or alcohol	7.5 mg sleep well							
Bedtime	10.45							
Lights out time	11.30							
Time taken to fall asleep	55 mins							
Number of times woke in the night	4							
Amount of time awake in the night	60 mins							
Final wake-up time	6.00							
Get up time	7.30							
Quality of sleep 0 = very poor sleep 10 = very good sleep	3							
Tinnitus annoyance 0 = no annoyance 10 = extremely annoying	7							
Time in bed	8 hrs 45 mins							
Total sleep time	4 hrs 35 mins							
Daytime functioning 0 = very poor 10 = no problems	7							

Record and evaluate your NATs about sleep and tinnitus

Also look carefully at your NATs about tinnitus and sleep. Follow the steps described in Chapter 7 for evaluating NATs. It can be difficult to 'catch' NATs, so here are the commonest sleep-related ones, which may give you a clue to your own.

- I won't sleep.
- I will be tormented all night.
- I will be exhausted tomorrow.
- I won't function well tomorrow.
- Bad sleep will damage my health.
- I will have a nervous breakdown.

In addition to these general NATs about sleep, it is common if you have tinnitus to hold the following NATs:

- Tinnitus will trouble me all night.
- My tinnitus will be worse tomorrow.
- The tinnitus will stop me sleeping.
- It will wake me up.

These lead to the other tinnitus-related NATs given in Chapter 7.

Once you have identified your NATs, ask yourself how they make you feel and whether or not you have changed your behaviour. Be careful to identify any 'middle of the night' thinking. Use the suggestions given for how to do this in Chapter 7 to help you evaluate your sleep-related NATs.

If you are able to tackle your NATs at night, all well and good, but it can be especially difficult to do this in the middle of the night. For this reason, people try to stop themselves thinking at such times. As shown in Chapter 9, however, trying to stop yourself thinking is usually counterproductive.

Sometimes it is possible to stop rumination by thinking about something else, though. When trying this in the middle of the night, it is best to focus on something that is not emotionally stimulating. For this reason, it can be helpful to repeat a single word over and over to reduce the flow of NATs through their mind. A word such as 'the' is suitable as it has no emotional meaning. You should actually say the word, silently, rather than just imagine it. If you can, keep saying it until you fall asleep. Alternatively, doing some mental arithmetic can help distract you. Start with 10,000 and take away 7 each time, for example. Another option is to focus on creating an image of a soothing scene. As before, the more detailed the image the better, so include sights, sounds, smells, touch and so on if you can.

Not all clinicians agree that these thought-blocking and distraction techniques are helpful in the long run. They can amount to safety behaviours, but do seem to provide some relief.

If you do use this approach, it is important that you think about your NATs again during the day. You may find that working on them in the day will cause them to have less impact at night. Because bedtime is the first point in the day that many of us stop doing things and are no longer distracted, it can be an opportunity for the mind to become very busy, so allow your mind to be busy on this *before* bedtime.

Set aside a short time (say 15 minutes, perhaps using a kitchen timer) during the day or early evening to sit and allow your thoughts to come to mind. You may find that the cares of the day or bigger worries pop into your head. It may be that you can't solve the problems there and then, but write them down on paper and reflect on the first steps you need to take to deal with them.

This planning or 'worry session' is unlikely to stop all thinking at other times, but it may reduce the impact of such thoughts at bedtime. If new ones intrude when you're in bed, refer them to the next day's worry session.

Reduce your levels of stress arousal

Relaxation exercises can play a helpful role in calming the body. They can also help calm the mind (see Chapter 8).

Generally, relaxation exercises are more helpful if you remain awake throughout them, but, if your main problem is poor sleep, do the exercises in bed and, if you fall asleep, that is a good result. Doing relaxation exercises also provides a better alternative to worry when you wake in the middle of the night.

Changes in behaviour

Once you have evaluated your NATs about sleep and tinnitus as best you can by writing them down and reflecting on their accuracy, it is time to think about your behaviour.

Work out what changes have taken place in how you do things. Do you do some things much more than before you had tinnitus? Do you do some things much less? Do you do some new things?

What changes you have made will depend on the content of your NATs and how you think you can keep safe from the predicted difficulties. There are, however, some common safety behaviours associated with sleep problems. Such changes in behaviour, listed below, can not only keep your NATs alive but also make your quality of sleep worse.

- *Behaviour that interferes with the sleep cycle* Sleeping late in the morning, getting as much sleep as possible during the day and at weekends, napping in the day, going to bed early, delaying going to bed.
- *Behaviour that interferes with getting to sleep* Drinking tea or coffee, planning for the next day, exercising late in the day, watching TV in bed, reading in bed.
- *Paradoxical fuelling of thoughts* Telling yourself to stop worrying, trying to stop thinking about problems, telling yourself to go to sleep quickly.
- *Behaviour that increases daytime sleepiness* Taking things easy, skipping exercise, cancelling work.
- *Behaviour that makes the day unpleasant or boring* Napping, avoiding people, slowing down the pace of the day, lowering your expectations of yourself, cancelling appointments, taking time off work.
- *Behaviour that keeps you preoccupied with sleep* Planning bedtime based on getting up time, calculating how much sleep you got, planning the day based on how much sleep you got, making plans for catching up on sleep.

You will notice that some of the changes relate to the things you do during the day. You may also have made changes that are connected specifically to your tinnitus. Usually these are connected to the use of sound enrichment. There is a fine line here between these changes being helpful and them amounting to safety behaviours, so you will need to make careful judgements about exactly how helpful they are to you (we discuss sound enrichment in more detail below).

If you do recognize any of the changes listed above, follow the steps given in Chapter 9 to change your behaviour. Ask yourself why you are doing them and connect them to your NATs. Work out what you could do differently that would test your worrying idea. This might involve doing something in another way or perhaps not doing something that you would usually. Once you've decided what to change, make a prediction about what will happen when you do so. Try things out and note exactly what does happen and consider what the outcome means for your original NAT.

Avoid checking and monitoring

Your anxieties about sleep will lead to you have selective attention about it. The most usual ways in which this happens is that you find yourself checking:

- your body for signs of falling asleep or being awake;
- the level of your tinnitus;
- the environment for signs of not falling asleep;
- the clock or your bedside sound generator to see how long it takes you to fall asleep;
- the clock to calculate how much sleep you will get;
- the clock in the morning, to see how many hours of sleep you got;
- your body during the day for signs of poor sleep or fatigue;
- your performance and functioning during the day.

Being aware that you are checking in these ways may help you do less of it. You can reduce your clockwatching by turning the face of the clock away from you. This allows you still to use the clock's alarm. Your sleep diary asks you to note things only at certain times and only briefly.

Behavioural management strategies

There are several general things that you can do to structure your day in ways that will make it easier for you to sleep.

- *Exercise* Fit people sleep better than unfit people. Exercise should be taken no later than the late afternoon or early evening, though, as exercise near bedtime may make it harder to fall asleep.
- *Food and drink* Snacks before bedtime should be light and drinks should be limited. Sticking to a routine helps. Avoid eating if you wake in the middle of the night, otherwise you might train yourself to be hungry in the night. Limit your intake of caffeine – coffee, tea, cola and so on – and alcohol. Although the latter will help you fall asleep, it disrupts the sleep cycle and makes sleep worse overall. Indeed, a regular heavy intake of alcohol can contribute to you feeling depressed and this will disrupt your sleep.
- *Bed is only for sleeping* Set a work or activity deadline, stopping 90 minutes before bedtime. Then go to bed and turn the lights out immediately. Do not read or watch TV in bed – these are activities you do when you're awake.
- *Go to bed when sleepy* Go then rather than at a set time out of habit.
- *Get up if you can't sleep* If you are not asleep about 25 minutes after going to bed, get up and sit in another room, doing something quiet and relaxing. You could read something soothing or do a relaxation exercise, for example. Then, go back to bed when you are sleepy again. Repeat if necessary.
- *Set your alarm for the same time every day* Do this even at weekends. Do not nap during the day and do not take recovery sleep to compensate for a previous bad night's sleep.

- *Do not try too hard to fall asleep* Tell yourself that sleep will come when it is ready and relaxing in bed is almost as good.
- *Don't stay in bed too long* It is very common for people who are worried about sleep to spend long periods of time in bed, much of it awake. Spending less time in bed can actually help to improve your sleep. Look at your sleep record and check how much sleep you actually get. Once you have worked this out, aim to spend only that amount of time in bed. For example, if, on average, you are getting five hours' sleep a night, spend only five hours in bed. Work out what time you need to get up and count backwards, so, if you need to get up at 6.30 a.m. and you typically get five hours' sleep, go to bed at 1.30 a.m. This sounds tough and it is! You are likely to be tired and want to go to bed. You may also find it hard to know what to do until that time of the night. The obvious things, such as reading and watching TV, might make you too sleepy. Some people save mundane housework tasks for this time as they are neither too stimulating nor sedating. This technique is called sleep restriction. You may even get less sleep to begin with, but it can lead to more continuous and satisfying sleep. You will probably need to keep it up for several weeks in order to see the benefits. Once your sleep has settled down and almost all the time you spend in bed is asleep (85 per cent of it), you can go to bed 15 minutes earlier. You can then make bedtime another 15 minutes earlier each time your sleep gets to 85 per cent of the time you spend in bed. Keeping careful records will help you know when to move on. This can be a very powerful technique if you can manage to keep it up. It is suitable if you are getting at least four hours' sleep a night.

Sound therapy at night

The use of sound can be of benefit if you have trouble sleeping.

Some people have the television or radio on, but this is not recommended as TV and radio programmes are designed to grab your attention. Instead, an inexpensive sound generator can deliver gentle sounds at night, by the bedside or via a pillow with a small speaker embedded inside.

The best sorts of sounds for this purpose are generally natural, including rain, the ocean and woods, though this is entirely a matter of personal choice. There is no magic sound. Once you have found a sound that is soothing and acceptable, it is best to leave the sound generator on that setting and not keep changing it.

It may be that your partner will find it hard to put up with the sounds that help you and even consider moving to another bedroom!

If this is the case, pillows that have a small speaker built into them or a speaker designed to work under the pillow can prove useful. Perhaps surprisingly, though, most people say that their partners find these sound generators acceptable or even pleasant.

The aim of sound therapy at night is to use quiet sounds to reduce the starkness of the tinnitus in a quiet environment and so promote better sleep. While some people like to use the device's timer, so that the sound is switched off after a set period, it is a good idea to leave it on all night. You may otherwise find yourself repeatedly switching the device on after the time period has elapsed, which can be disruptive in itself and keep you focused on your sleep problem. Also, because even a normal night's sleep involves a number of awakenings, leaving the device on will mean that you do not wake up in the middle of the night in a very quiet room. Likewise, it may reduce the starkness of your tinnitus on waking in the morning.

Some clinicians suggest leaving the device on 24 hours a day, which removes the unhappy bedtime routine of switching it on and makes it easier to get used to sound in the bedroom. If so, it makes economical sense to invest in one that has a mains adaptor rather than batteries. It also allows you to ignore the device, which means you focus less on your tinnitus.

Should I take sleeping pills?

In the UK, the National Institute for Health and Clinical Excellence (NICE, at <www.nice.org.uk>), in its publication on insomnia (NICE, 2004), suggests that sleeping pills such as benzodiazepines (for example, Temazepam and the newer 'Z medicines' (zopiclone, zaleplon and so on) can be very helpful in promoting sleep if used for a short period of time. They should not be used for longer, though, because people tend to develop a tolerance of them (which means that more of them need to be taken to have the same effect or they stop working) or dependence on them.

Sometimes people have withdrawal symptoms when they stop using benzodiazepines, which can include tinnitus. Long-term use of sleeping pills can actually make sleep problems worse and these drugs don't treat the underlying causes.

The NICE guidelines suggest that psychological techniques such as those outlined in this chapter be used for the treatment of insomnia.

Mary experienced some sleep problems. Here is how she dealt with them.

Mary

Mary believed that it took her up to two hours to fall asleep and that she woke an hour and a half later, when it would take her up to an hour to get back to sleep again. While awake, her attention was captured by worries about the loss of sleep and her tinnitus.

Mary believed it was her tinnitus that prevented her from sleeping and the loss of sleep was a sign she was having a nervous breakdown. The time she spent resting on the sofa during the day and the reduction in her general activity level was partly to compensate for what she believed would be the bad effects of her sleep loss – that is, an inability to function normally and a slide into mental illness.

Keeping a careful sleep log helped Mary to see that her sleep was actually slightly better than she thought. Finding out more about her sleep helped her understand that her difficulty was the result of a busy mind rather than just the fact that she had tinnitus.

As a result, early in the evenings, Mary now spends 15 minutes allowing her worrying thoughts to come into her mind and then she uses a thought-blocking technique while awake in bed. This has reduced the strength of her thoughts when in bed.

Mary has also reduced the amount of time she spends resting during the day and increased her general activity levels, which has helped reduce her concerns that her sleep problems were leading to a nervous breakdown. It has also allowed her to use energy during the day and improved the regulation of her sleep cycle. Mary has also found a bedside sound generator helpful.

Some final thoughts

The message we would like you to take away from this chapter is that, although many people who have troublesome tinnitus have difficulty sleeping, this is not inevitable. Lots of people with tinnitus, even troublesome tinnitus, sleep well. The things that interfere with sleep are worry, stress arousal and changes in behaviour (including daytime behaviour) rather than tinnitus per se. Sleep is a busy process and requires careful examination, but, if your sleep is bad, following the guidelines we have set out here should help to make a difference.

12

Moving on and avoiding relapse

Being able to stand back from your thoughts and evaluate them, rather than simply accept them, seems to be of particular importance in ensuring that you don't get sucked into vicious circles some time in the future. In other words, the ability to think about your thinking can be protective against future emotional storms.

This is referred to as the ability to *decentre* from your thoughts and sometimes known by the technical name *meta-cognitive insight*. It involves being able to recognize your thoughts as just that rather than necessarily representing reality. Being able to view negative thoughts and feelings as passing events that may or may not have some truth in them makes it less likely that you will be swept along in a whirlwind of emotion by the next stressful event, whether this is a change in your tinnitus or anything else.

There are various approaches that can help you to develop meta-cognitive insight. One is to repeatedly carry out the exercises referred to in Chapters 7, 8 and 9. Another is *mindfulness meditation*, which helps you to be aware of what is happening to you without judging or fighting it. There is evidence that this kind of meditation is helpful in managing depression and a number of medical conditions, most notably chronic pain. At the time of writing, this approach is being used in a few tinnitus clinics and the evidence for its benefits is emerging.

If you would like to try this approach and your local audiology department does not yet offer it, you may find that general classes are available at your local community centre or Buddhist centre (it is not necessary to be a Buddhist to take part).

For some, the journey of recovery from tinnitus can involve many ups and downs. If you have been making progress and feel bad again, it is easy to believe that you are back to square one. It is also possible for things to seem worse before they get better. Figure 12.1 (overleaf) shows the sort of ups and downs that are typical of many people's progress.

Remember, having tinnitus does not give you immunity from the rest of life's events, such as bereavement, financial crises, relationship problems or other unrelated illness. Tinnitus can act as an emotional barometer. As you become more stressed, your resources for coping

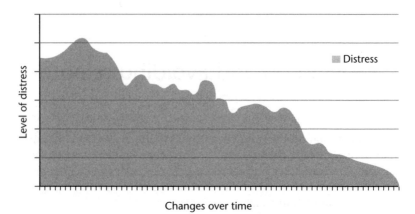

Figure 12.1 The ups and downs typical of many people's recovery from the distress of their tinnitus

become more stretched and the result is that the tinnitus becomes more intrusive. There may also be natural variations in your mood that can make it seem like a setback is happening for no reason. While none of us knows what awaits us in life, there are some tactics that can help reduce the likelihood of a relapse.

Preventing relapse

The first thing to do is take care of yourself. It is easy, for example, to slip into poor patterns of working. Perhaps a crisis at work leads you to make an extraordinary effort, then that becomes expected of you (by yourself or others) on an ongoing basis.

Having a good work–life balance is important for us all, which includes investing time and effort in hobbies or other things that enrich us. Our own interests include painting, woodcarving and studying theology (though not all at the same time!) and we commend finding absorbing pastimes if you have tinnitus.

While old ideas about diet and tinnitus have largely been discounted, having a balanced, healthy diet is an important element in maintaining good general health and it is easier to deal with your tinnitus if you are generally well. Common sense dictates taking care regarding your alcohol intake. Keeping active and fit also make sense, though for some with tinnitus there is a temptation to exercise obsessively, which is a pitfall to avoid.

Another positive thing you can do sometimes is to reflect on your journey into recovery. This doesn't need to be deep navel gazing, but just pausing to consider how much recovery you have made and how it was supported by some relatively commonsense actions.

What should I do if I do relapse?

First, deal with the situation that has triggered the relapse. If it is a bereavement or relationship breakdown, consider seeking counselling. If your finances triggered it, seek debt advice from, for example, in the UK, the Citizens Advice Bureau.

Then, methodically and carefully, go back to the tactics that helped you recover previously. It is common sense to say that if you managed it once, you will again. Put back in place the combination of relaxation, sound therapy and understanding that was of benefit initially.

Reviewing your situation with your tinnitus clinician can also be useful. In the UK, this may take some time to arrange, but it is the practice of many tinnitus clinicians to place past patients on an 'SOS' list, whereby they can re-access the clinic without delay.

Summary

As with many other situations in life, progress can be a case of two steps forward, one step back. When a setback seems to be happening, taking care to revisit both your understanding of your situation and the positive strategies that have supported you in the past can be very effective in resuming your progress towards recovery.

13

Helping other people with tinnitus

It is possible that you're reading this not because you have tinnitus, but a friend or family member has it. In this chapter, we look at how you can help adults and children, so take from the following advice what will help your own particular situation.

Helping adults you know who have tinnitus

Do read the rest of this book to become more knowledgeable about tinnitus and hyperacusis, as this will help throw some light on what your friend or relative is going through.

Companionship

Someone with tinnitus can feel very lonely and isolated. As we saw in Chapter 6, tinnitus can cause people to withdraw. Just having someone else around can be therapeutic and, for some, this is especially true during the night as it is their worst time.

Avoid apportioning blame

It is quite possible that you feel, or indeed the person with tinnitus feels, that he or she has brought the problem on him- or herself – if it started after a visit to a noisy nightclub, for example. 'If only . . .' statements can then become very common: 'If only you hadn't gone to the nightclub', 'If only we could turn back time.'

Such thinking is understandable, but unhelpful and more likely to lead to conflict than a solution. In any case, they are usually incorrect. Taking the example of the nightclub, for example, exposure to noise can certainly help to trigger tinnitus, but is rarely the only factor. The vast majority of people who go to nightclubs do not develop persistent tinnitus.

It is also possible to blame someone else's tinnitus for impinging negatively on your own life. You may feel, for instance, that your friend or relative's tinnitus is preventing you from doing things that you want to do. You might like to go on holiday, but he or she is scared that the noise or pressure changes associated with flying in an aeroplane may worsen the tinnitus. As a result, you can end up resenting the tinnitus for its impact on you. Try to avoid this pitfall as most of these life restrictions are temporary.

Take an interest in the problem

Because there are no outward signs of tinnitus or hyperacusis, it is easy to forget that someone has these problems. Consequently, many people with the symptoms feel that they are being ignored by those around them. So, asking about the tinnitus periodically can help the person you know open up and discuss his or her difficulties.

There is, however, a major caveat to this advice: do be tactful. Repeatedly asking questions about the tinnitus can be counterproductive as it can cause the person to focus more on the tinnitus than is helpful or simply become irritated with you for asking the questions.

Help with treatments

Many people with tinnitus or hyperacusis feel that there is no point in them seeking help, but everyone with tinnitus should have, at the very least, a medical check-up and hearing test. You can help by persuading your friend or relative to visit the doctor.

You can also offer to accompany him or her to the appointment. Various studies have shown that people only remember a small fraction of what doctors tell them, so it is useful to have two sets of ears taking in information during the consultation. This is especially true if the person has some kind of hearing loss.

Some treatments can affect people other than the person with tinnitus, too. Occasionally this is the case with sound therapy, for example (see Chapter 10).

If you are the partner of someone using a sound generator, you may worry that this will interfere with your own sleep. Perhaps surprisingly, this is usually not the case. In fact, many people without tinnitus sleep better if there is some quiet sound in the bedroom. We have even supplied sound generators to people who do not have tinnitus! If this is you, we would therefore strongly advise you to set aside your preconceptions and give it a go. If you really do find that it is disturbing your sleep, there are pillows with built-in speakers or flat loudspeakers that are placed underneath a pillow so that only the person with tinnitus hears the sound.

People with tinnitus and any associated hearing loss are often advised to try a hearing aid. Some people are reluctant, pointing out that their major problem is a horrible noise inside their head, not a difficulty with hearing.

You can help in this situation by being reassuring and pointing out that hearing aids can help by allowing him or her to concentrate more on external sounds than the internal tinnitus.

Some people with tinnitus find it helpful to attend self-help groups so that they can meet other people with the same difficulties that they have. Again, offering to accompany them is helpful, especially for the initial visits.

Avoid endless searching

Some people are constantly on the lookout for any new treatments that will help their friend or relative. They are always cutting articles out of newspapers or printing material from the Internet. We advise against this.

It is very natural for you to feel powerless about the problem and desperately want to help and provide a solution. Unfortunately, repeatedly raising someone's hopes and expectations, only to have those hopes dashed, is dispiriting and counterproductive.

Journalists understandably tend to make their articles seem as exciting and interesting as possible. They therefore provide details of the newest treatments and frequently put a very positive slant on the information. Closer scientific scrutiny, though, often shows that the so-called 'treatment' is actually at a very experimental stage, has significant drawbacks and is only applicable to a small number of people. If there is a genuine breakthrough in the treatment of tinnitus, it will become public knowledge in a very short space of time. You will not have to scour the deepest reaches of the World Wide Web to find a solution.

Carry on life as normally as possible

As discussed in Chapter 6, tinnitus can restrict people's lives. Do encourage your friend or relative to try and maintain as normal a life as possible, without being forceful. Rekindling interest in previous hobbies can be helpful and, if he or she is spiritual, encouraging him or her to maintain this is beneficial.

Patience

Improvements in tinnitus can be a slow process, with many ups and downs. This is normal, so do not expect dramatic progress and become disheartened when there are dips or it seems to take ages before something positive happens.

Look after yourself

You can only help someone else if you are in a good state yourself. It is possible for someone's tinnitus to drag down those around them. Make sure this does not happen to you, by, for example, allowing yourself to have some time away from the problem. In some situations, where the impact of the tinnitus or hyperacusis has been severe, you might benefit from having some supportive counselling.

Helping children with tinnitus and hyperacusis

Optimism

The first thing to say about tinnitus in children is that it is usually less of a problem than tinnitus in adults.

Although children are commonly aware of their tinnitus, it does not seem to cause them distress into adulthood. Also, the majority of children with tinnitus spontaneously recover. So, it is unusual to see adults with tinnitus who say that they have had a problem since childhood.

Children are much more adaptable than adults. In scientific jargon, their brains display great plasticity. They are therefore much more able than adults to adjust to new sensations and, hence, can tune out their tinnitus.

This is not to belittle tinnitus in childhood – it can be a real problem – but the chances of improvement are excellent so having a positive outlook is both valid and helpful.

Can the advice given in this book be applied to children?

Much of this book is based on the psychological treatment called cognitive behavioural therapy (CBT). This can be undertaken with children as well as adults, but using language that is appropriate to the child's age. It can, however, be more complicated when working with children, so it is advisable to seek expert help. This is probably one of those occasions when self-help is not always appropriate.

Other therapies that are discussed, such as sound therapy, can be applied in childhood in a very similar way to that used in adulthood.

Taking an interest and being reassuring

Children with tinnitus and hyperacusis can feel just as isolated and lonely as adults and benefit from being able to talk about their symptoms. Young children will use very different language to explain their symptoms, so you will need to tune in to their way of thinking.

Children are very good at picking up subtle messages from those around them, so, if you are anxious or worried about your child's tinnitus, that anxiety can all too easily be transferred to him or her. It is much better if you adopt a positive and reassuring manner.

Avoid apportioning blame

Just as with adults, it is important not to suggest that children with tinnitus have brought the problem on themselves.

Help with treatments

Unlike in adulthood, tinnitus in childhood is slightly more likely to have an underlying cause, such as migraine. It is therefore important that a child with tinnitus should have a medical assessment.

One problem that parents encounter is that there are very few healthcare professionals who are experienced and comfortable dealing with childhood tinnitus. You may need considerable patience and perseverance to find such a person.

Children generally like to fit in with their peers and not seem different or unusual. If they are advised to wear hearing aids or wearable sound generators (see Chapter 10) this can cause them significant worry. You can help by offering support and reassurance.

Carry on life as normally as possible

A lot of childhood activities either directly involve noise or happen in noisy environments – playing musical instruments, going to clubs, sporting events, concerts and activity centres can all be noisy. It can be devastating, therefore, for a child to find that such noise worsens their tinnitus or an activity becomes intolerable due to their hyperacusis.

Sound-attenuating earplugs can allow children with tinnitus or hyperacusis to attend noisy functions, but care should be taken to not overdo their usage. If earplugs are worn too much and in situations where the noise levels are not excessive, it can cause the auditory system to become more sensitive, which can worsen the tinnitus or hyperacusis. In other words, you should only let children use sound-attenuating earplugs when it is genuinely noisy.

School

School can be a challenging place for children with tinnitus or hyperacusis. These conditions can interfere with their ability to concentrate on their schoolwork, which can result in them being labelled inattentive, lazy or worse. School can also be noisy – playground noise, assemblies, sport and even the use of bells to mark the ends of lessons, breaks and lunchtime can all temporarily increase the intrusiveness of tinnitus and hyperacusis. Conversely, school can also involve quite a lot of time sitting in very quiet environments, which can make the tinnitus seem louder, especially when contrasted with noisy periods of time.

As discussed previously, stress tends to worsen both tinnitus and hyperacusis and school can be a very stressful place, particularly around the time of important examinations and tests.

You can help your child by explaining the nature of the problem to teaching staff. If necessary give them a copy of this book! Once they understand the condition, they can adapt your child's routine accordingly. For example, he or she may be better doing exams in a separate room where there is some gentle background sound rather than in the overwhelming quietness of an examination hall.

Similarly, children with tinnitus may occasionally need to have a few minutes' break from normal school activities if their tinnitus becomes intrusive. Also, if they are falling behind educationally, it is sensible to involve the special needs team as soon as possible (in the UK, this can be accomplished by contacting the school's special educational needs coordinator, or SENCO).

Above all, you should try to encourage your child to take as full and active a part in school as possible. Tinnitus and hyperacusis should not be used as an excuse for staying at home or avoiding various activities.

Home

One of the common difficulties arising from childhood tinnitus is that it often seems to result in sleep problems.

Sound generators (see Chapter 10) can be used. Other more innovative sound sources can also be used, such as the ticking of a clock, story CDs, the bubbling of a fish tank or the whirr of a fan. Some such sounds can also be used if your child finds their tinnitus is intrusive while doing their homework. Alternatively, quiet background music can be played in these situations, but you should be quite firm that the music is there to *facilitate* homework, not as an alternative to doing the homework.

Patience

Just as with adults, making improvements can be a slow process, with many ups and downs. This is normal and you should not expect dramatic positive changes to occur.

Summary

It can be very difficult seeing someone you care for struggle with tinnitus or hyperacusis. Being positive and supportive is important, but this can only be really effective if you understand the situation and how recovery can be possible.

Appendix: Tinnitus mechanisms

In this appendix we discuss some of the scientific theories that have been put forward to try and explain exactly what is going on in the ears, auditory nerve and brain.

Background neural activity

In Chapter 2, we mentioned that it has been found that even people without tinnitus can hear tinnitus-like sounds when they listen carefully in silence.

The theory is that, in this situation, they are aware of background electrical activity in their hearing nerve which would usually be masked by external sounds. Experiments have shown that this is because the hearing nerve, rather than being passive in the way that a copper wire is, is actually constantly and randomly active. This isn't normally perceived as it is at a low level, not organized into a pattern and constantly present, so the brain filters it out (this, you will recall, is the process called habituation). In contrast, when we hear an external sound, a pattern is imposed on the randomness and that gives the brain a signal to listen to.

The development of tinnitus may involve changes in the awareness of this background activity. The arguments for this are strongest concerning people with normal hearing who have tinnitus.

One suggestion is that the background activity may increase as it does seem to be influenced by certain brain chemicals called neurotransmitters (specifically, one called glutamate) and some drugs.

Another proposal is that the background random activity becomes more organized, so it appears to signal a sound to the brain. This synchronization has been induced in laboratory experiments, but has not yet been proven in clinics.

Finally, it is possible that the level of awareness of the sound may change. Thus, someone who was previously unaware of it becomes able to hear this background noise. Certainly, anxiety and stress change our awareness of our senses and we can become more vigilant than normal to new sensations at such times.

The role of the cochlea (the inner ear)

For many years, tinnitus research focused almost exclusively on the possibility that the cochlea is involved in the ignition of tinnitus. As described in Chapter 2, the cochlea is an intricate, sensitive and fragile organ concerned with converting the physical energy of sound into patterns of activity in the nerve of hearing that the brain can interpret. Its fragile structure makes the cochlea prone to damage, whether this is by drugs, noise or disease.

Several ideas have been proposed concerning the contribution cochlear dysfunction makes to tinnitus. A traditional view is that when cochlear hair cells are damaged, they send distorted, spontaneous signals to the brain that are interpreted as sound, so causing tinnitus. This led to analogies being made such as a doorbell that is stuck and keeps ringing.

This idea, however, no longer appears to be supported by evidence. When a mammal loses its hearing there is, in fact, a decrease in spontaneous signals from the cochlea to the brain rather than the increase predicted by this view. The one exception seems to be cochlear hair cell damage due to noise, where an increase in spontaneous firing can be observed in experiments. This has led to theories that noise-induced tinnitus may be due to outer hair cell (OHC) dysfunction, these cells being more vulnerable to noise damage than the inner hair cells (IHC).

A role of the OHC in the onset of tinnitus has also been claimed by researchers studying the effect of large doses of aspirin (acetylsalicylic acid) on the cochlea. There is a temporary dysfunction of the OHC, which affects the fine-tuning process of hearing, resulting in hearing loss and tinnitus, both of which usually resolve after the drug has been metabolized.

The doses needed for this to happen, though, are massively in excess of those taken for either pain relief or to prevent heart attacks and stroke. The same effects can be seen when quinine is given, but, again, the effect is usually temporary and the dosage required is much greater than that usually used for the prevention of malaria or cramps.

Another suggestion regarding the role of these hair cells in tinnitus involves the relationship between the OHC and IHC. As mentioned above, the OHC are more vulnerable than the IHC, so there can be a situation where the OHC are physically damaged and the IHC are intact. This situation has been called *discordant damage*.

It has been suggested, therefore, that the OHC would not be able to support the membrane above them, which would drop down on to the IHC below and these would fire off impulses to the brain. An analogy would be a tent full of Scouts. If the tent pole (OHC) broke, the tent would drop down on to the Scouts (IHC), who would react by being very energetic!

This theory predicts that if someone has a hearing loss that means he or she cannot hear high-frequency sounds, plus associated tinnitus, the pitch of that tinnitus will be just at the frequency of the sounds the person can no longer hear as that will be the area of discordant damage. In some patients this is the case, though by no means in all, so this theory is not universally accepted.

The function of the cochlear hair cells in converting sound from vibrational energy into a pattern of neural activity that the brain can interpret is complex and involves many biochemical and metabolic processes. One that has been mentioned as a cause of tinnitus relates to the role calcium plays in the functioning of the hair cells.

There is evidence to indicate that higher concentrations of calcium in the cochlear fluids that surround the hair cells can cause an increase in the rate of spontaneous firing of the auditory nerve. This would result in an increase in the background noise in the hearing system, which might be heard as tinnitus.

As mentioned above, researchers have investigated why there is a link between large doses of aspirin and tinnitus. They have noted that overdoses of the drug can cause a change in the amount of calcium in the hair cells, but also that it activates a specific type of receptor in the auditory nerve at the base of these cells. These receptors are called N-methyl-D-aspartate (NMDA) and such activity would cause spontaneous activity in the auditory nerve.

This is of some interest, as NMDA receptors also seem to be activated during periods of stress – in this latter situation by increased levels of the neurotransmitter glutamate. The fact that many people with tinnitus find it is exacerbated by stress has led scientists to propose it may be due to the role of the NMDA receptors, so work is ongoing to improve our knowledge in this area.

Changes in hearing after injury

For many years, it was believed that the human nervous system could not recover after injury. Then, the opposite was proposed by a Spanish neuro-anatomist called Ramón y Cajal (1852–1934), who had suggested that the recovery observed after injury and the ability of humans to learn new skills implies that the nervous system is actually able to change quite dramatically.

This was very controversial and, indeed, it is only quite recently that it has come to be accepted by the mainstream and been applied to the auditory system, too.

The important idea to grasp here is that the nervous system is *plastic* – that is, it can change – and it can *reorganize* – functions can be resited within the brain. The implication is that, after a change in the sensitivity of the cochlea causing a hearing loss, there are changes in the auditory system within the brain, which reorganizes the available processing power to maximize the hearing of those frequencies that are still picked up by the cochlea. This occurs when there are both slow gradual changes, as in age-related hearing loss, and sudden changes, which can occur as a result of a virus attacking the cochlea, following surgery or an injury.

Experiments have indicated that the reorganization can be rapid (taking a period of a few weeks) and very sizeable. It can be imperfect, however, leading to areas of the brain that are spontaneously active, especially at the edges or boundaries of the reorganized areas. In the parts of the brain involved in hearing, such spontaneous bursting activity would be perceived as sound and this may underlie some people's experiences of tinnitus.

The emotional system

To focus purely on the auditory areas of the brain is insufficient, however, to achieve an understanding of hearing and, indeed, tinnitus. There are connections between the auditory areas of the brain and those concerned with emotion and attention to sound at many levels.

Neuroscientists draw together the various structures within the brain involved with emotion under the title *the limbic system*. The hearing pathways feed into various parts of this limbic system, which explains why sound can cause massive emotional responses. An example would be listening to music, which can give us great feelings of awe and beauty. In this situation, the music stimulates and interfaces directly with the limbic system, causing such deep feelings. Similarly, the sounds people with tinnitus hear directly stimulate emotions, which, as we saw in Chapter 2, can be apprehension and even fear. The point that we make in this book, however, is that this can be changed.

Reacting to sound

We can be agitated, alerted or startled by sounds far more readily than is the case with smells, touch or visual input. In our everyday lives our phones, computers, microwaves, alarm clocks and doorbells all bleep and ring at us and we attend to them without delay.

Evolutionary biologists believe this is an indication that hearing in mammals has long functioned as a way of detecting danger. By attending to new sounds in the environment, we can identify those that might mean there is a danger or threat; this raises our levels of arousal and agitation, causing the 'fight or flight' response described earlier.

The Jastreboff neurophysiological model

A way of understanding these aspects of the experience of tinnitus was suggested by Professor Pawel Jastreboff – a neuroscientist of Polish origin now working in the USA. He drew together various ideas that were circulating about tinnitus into a model to give us a way of understanding how they fit together.

In the Jastreboff neurophysiological model (JNM), it is proposed that tinnitus usually has its origin in the cochlear or auditory nerve (though it can be higher in the brain) and it is detected in the auditory centres in the brainstem, which is the part of the brain that regulates activities such as breathing, eating and sleeping. Connections at this low level within the brain with systems of reaction and emotion set up a loop of reaction, agitation and distress.

This understanding of tinnitus places much more emphasis on these lower brain functions than the higher functions of meaning, belief, personality and experience. Although the JNM is attractive, there have been some criticisms, particularly regarding the focus on lower brain functions but also because the model suggests that tinnitus develops as a result of a sequence of conditioned responses. This last is a simple kind of learning that humans certainly can do, but we usually learn and develop behaviours by more complex means.

A psychological model

The way in which tinnitus becomes troublesome had been considered before the work of Pawel Jastreboff by a team of clinicians and researchers working at the Royal National Throat, Nose & Ear Hospital in London, UK. The team included both medical doctors and psychologists, but their work is often called the psychological model of tinnitus as it carefully considers the roles of attention and emotion in the development of tinnitus-related distress.

The model put forward the idea that, as someone becomes aware of tinnitus, the auditory system focuses on it – the technical term for this being that it produces an *orienting response*. A reaction occurs, involving alertness and agitation, and even greater vigilance is given over to the tinnitus.

It was predicted that this situation would be more likely to develop if:

- the tinnitus had a strong emotional component, possibly because it resulted from injury or failed surgery or it was thought of as threatening;
- the tinnitus had particularly unpleasant qualities;
- the person was already agitated, alert and vigilant, perhaps due to stress.

While the proponents of the Jastreboff neurophysiological and the psychological models of tinnitus have not come to an agreement, careful consideration of these two perspectives leads us to conclude that, while they are not in total agreement, there are substantial areas of convergence. They both suggest that people normally habituate to their tinnitus, they both highlight the observation that people's emotional reactions are a key factor when habituation is slow to occur and they both suggest methods for minimizing those reactions.

Resources

Compared with the situation a few years ago, there is now a wealth of information about tinnitus and hyperacusis available to the public. Care needs to be taken with information from the Internet, and messageboards in particular, but the resources given below should help you.

General self-help and peer support

There are several strong and active peer support groups for people with troublesome tinnitus and hyperacusis, in the UK and elsewhere.

UK

British Tinnitus Association
Ground Floor, Unit 5
Acorn Business Park
Woodseats Close
Sheffield S8 0TB
Tel.: 0114 250 9922 (general); 0800 018 0527 (free helpline)
Website: www.tinnitus.org.uk

Royal National Institute for Deaf People
19–23 Featherstone Street
London EC1Y 8SL
Tel.: 0808 808 0123; textphone: 0808 808 9000 (both freephone information lines)
Website: www.rnid.org.uk/shop/products/tinnitus

It is generally thought that devices for tinnitus are more effective if issued in a clinic by professionals, with clear instructions and objectives for their use. However, some people will not be able to access specialist clinical services, and so will need to buy devices independently. RNID's large online shop provides a catalogue with a large range of items including table-top sound generators and sound pillows. Ear-level sound generators are available via <www.amazon.co.uk>. As with all online shopping, a cautious approach should be taken.

Overseas

American Tinnitus Association
Website: www.ata.org

German Tinnitus League
Website: www.tinnitus-liga.de

Hyperacusis Network
Website: www.hyperacusis.net

Irish Tinnitus Association
35 North Frederick Street
Dublin 1
Tel.: 353 (0)1 817 5700
Website: www.deafhear.ie

Tinnitus Association of Canada
Website: www.kadis.com/ta/tinnitus.htm

Tinnitus South Australia
Website: www.tinnitussa.org

Research

While the tinnitus associations listed above will convey some information about research, a relatively recent and comprehensive source of information is the Tinnitus Research Initiative, based in the University of Regensburg in Germany <www. tinnitusresearch.org>. While the information is intended for professionals, it is clearly laid out and described.

Specific approaches

British Association for Behavioural and Cognitive Psychotherapies
Imperial House
Hornby Street
Bury BL9 5BN
Tel.: 0161 705 4304
Fax: 0161 705 4306
Website: www.babcp.com

Cognitive behavioural therapy (CBT) can help you manage your tinnitus and hyperacusis. Qualified CBT therapists can be found through this organization.

Tinnitus and Hyperacusis Centre
32 Devonshire Place
London W1G 6JB
Tel.: 020 7847 2701
Website: www.tinnitus.org

This centre specializes in Tinnitus Retraining Therapy (TRT), whose pioneers, Pawel Jastreboff and Jonathan Hazell, have been very open to sharing information about their ideas on the Web. They also suggest the use of CBT to help manage tinnitus and hyperacusis. The website has not been extensively updated for some time, but still contains a clear introduction to TRT.

Devices

It is generally advisable to have devices for tinnitus issued in a clinic by professionals, with clear instructions and objectives for their use, but, if you are unable to access such services, it is possible to buy them independently. If you do, exercise caution and reread the earlier chapters for some general guidelines on their use.

Royal National Institute for Deaf People
www.rnid.org.uk/shop/products/tinnitus

Sells a range of table-top sound generators and sound pillows.

Amazon
www.amazon.co.uk

Ear-level sound generators for tinnitus are available from the website.

Further reading

Tinnitus

Andersson, G., Baguley, D. M., McKenna, L., McFerran, D., *Tinnitus: A multidisciplinary approach*. Wiley-Blackwell, Oxford, 2005.
All the current approaches are described and the tinnitus literature reviewed.

Jastreboff, P. and Hazell, J. W. P., *Tinnitus Retraining Therapy*. Cambridge University Press, Cambridge, 2004.
Recently reissued in paperback, but not revised, this is the introduction to TRT for professionals, but is accessible to the lay reader.

Tyler, R. (ed.), *The Consumer Handbook on Tinnitus*, Auricle Ink Publishers, Sedona, Ariz., 2008.
A collection of chapters written by leading tinnitus specialists and covering a range of subjects.

Cognitive behavioural therapy

Burns, D., *The Feeling Good Handbook*, Plume, New York, 1999.
Butler, G. and Hope, T., *Manage Your Mind*, Oxford University Press, Oxford, 1995.
Cole, F., Macdonald, H., Carus, C. and Howden-Leach, H., *Overcoming Chronic Pain: A self-help guide using cognitive-behavioural techniques*, Constable & Robinson, London, 2005.
Fennell, M., *Overcoming Low Self-esteem: A self-help guide using cognitive-behavioural techniques*, Constable & Robinson, London, 1999.
Gilbert, P., *Overcoming Depression: A self-help guide using cognitive-behavioural techniques* (revised edition), Constable & Robinson, London, 2005.
Padesky, C. A. and Greenberg, D., *Clinician's Guide to Mind Over Mood*, Guilford Press, New York, 1995.
Kennerley, H., *Overcoming Anxiety: A self-help guide using cognitive-behavioural techniques*, Constable & Robinson, London, 1997.
Willson, R. and Branch, R., *Cognitive Behavioural Therapy for Dummies*, John Wiley & Sons, Chichester, 2006.

Sleep

Espie, C., *Overcoming Insomnia and Sleep Problems: A self-help guide using cognitive-behavioural techniques*, Constable & Robinson, London, 2006.

Horn, J., *Sleepfaring: A journey through the science of sleep*, Oxford University Press, Oxford, 2006.

National Institute for Health and Clinical Excellence, *Zaleplon, Zolpiden and Zopiclone for Insomnia: Understanding NICE guidance – information for people with insomnia, their families and carers, and the public*, NICE, London, 2004.

Mindfulness meditation

Kabat-Zinn, J., *Full Catastrophe Living: Using the wisdom of your body and mind to face stress, pain and illness*, Delta, New York, 1990.

Williams, M., Teasdale, J., Segal, Z. and Kabat-Zinn, J., *The Mindful Way through Depression: Freeing yourself from chronic unhappiness*, Guilford Press, New York, 2007.

Index